YMCA Healthy Back Book

YMCA of the USA

with Patricia Sammann

Human Kinetics Publishers

Library of Congress Cataloging-in-Publication Data

YMCA Healthy Back Book
    YMCA of the USA / Patricia Sammann.
         p.   cm.
    Includes index.
    ISBN 0-87322-629-1
    1. Backache–Popular works. 2. Backache–Exercise therapy.
  I. Title.
    RD771.B217S255 1994
    617.5'64–dc20   93-31736
                                               CIP

ISBN: 0-87322-629-1

Developmental Editor: Larret Galasyn-Wright; **Assistant Editor and Proofreader:** Dawn Roselund; **Copyeditor:** Christine Drews; **Indexer**: Theresa J. Schaefer; **Production Director:** Ernie Noa; **Keyboarder:** Kathleen Boudreau-Fuoss; **Book Designer and Illustrator:** Doug Burnett; **Cover Designer:** Keith Blomberg; **Medical Illustrator:** Anne Irène Hurley; **Printer:** Bang Printing.

Human Kinetics books are available at special discounts for bulk purchase. Special editions or book excerpts can also be created to specification. For details, contact the Special Sales Manager at Human Kinetics.

Printed in the United States of America

10 9 8 7 6 5 4 3 2 1

Human Kinetics Publishers
Box 5076, Champaign, IL 61825-5076
1-800-747-4457

Canada: Human Kinetics Publishers, Box 24040,
Windsor, ON N8Y 4Y9
1-800-465-7301 (in Canada only)

Europe: Human Kinetics Publishers (Europe) Ltd.,
P.O. Box IW14, Leeds LS16 6TR, England
0532-781708

Australia: Human Kinetics Publishers, P.O. Box 80,
Kingswood 5062, South Australia
618-374-0433

New Zealand: Human Kinetics Publishers, P.O. Box 105-231,
Auckland 1
(09) 309-2259

C O N T E N T S

Preface iv

Introduction: You Are Not Alone vi

Chapter 1   First Aid and Pain Relief for
Back Attacks   1

Chapter 2   Medical Help for Your Back   9

Chapter 3   How Your Back Works and
Why It Sometimes Doesn't   21

Chapter 4   Getting Your Back on Track
With Exercise   35

Chapter 5   Working With Your Back—
Not Against It   71

Chapter 6   A Healthy Lifestyle,
A Healthy Back   83

Acknowledgments 106

Credits 107

Index 108

Today, millions of people in the U.S. have chronic or acute back pain that requires professional treatment. And as our population ages, it's likely that even more people will experience back pain. The extent of the suffering ranges from slight twinges now and then to flat-on-your-back, immobilizing pain. Almost all of these people would like to find a cure.

Since 1974 the Y's guided exercise and education classes have brought relief from back pain to those who once were afraid to exercise because of their pain. Because back pain is so prevalent, the YMCA of the USA decided to attack it with a new national program designed to help every person with back pain not only reduce the pain but become healthier at the same time. They created a series of classes that teach each participant how to avoid further back pain, how to exercise to reduce the likelihood of pain, and how to reduce pain when it occurs. Best of all, the program places back care in the context of activities that promote better health.

The Y classes are based on the content of this book plus an additional, less strenuous level of exercises. If you are in a Y class, you have an instructor who can guide you through the information, answer your questions, and check that you learn to perform exercises and daily living tasks safely. You also have the advantage of sharing your learning experience with other people with back pain. But even if you're not in a Y class, this book can be your personal handbook to better back health. It's designed to present the information you need in an easy-to-understand format.

We begin this book by outlining the extent of back problems in America and its costs to our society. Chapter 1 then takes us to the issue at hand. You're probably reading this book because your back hurts. In chapter 1 we answer your questions about when to see a doctor and how to get relief at home. If you're in severe pain, you'll appreciate the first-aid kit the chapter provides.

You might decide you need medical help. Chapter 2 guides you in choosing a practitioner and preparing for the office visit. It also describes the treatment options you might be offered. In chapter 3 we provide a clear explanation of how the back works, with helpful illustrations that demonstrate the concepts. After we've listed the possible causes of back and neck pain, you can take a quiz to identify the most important controllable risk factors that may be causing your pain.

Exercises to help condition your back—and the rest of your body—make up chapter 4. Three levels of exercise allow you to start to exercise easily and to gradually work up to a 20-minute workout. We'll also encourage you to start aerobic activity if you don't already swim, bike, do low-impact aerobics, or enjoy other physical indoor and outdoor pursuits.

And if you think exercise isn't for you because of your physical limitations, think again! Chapter 4 also presents aquatic back exercises. If you would like to take advantage of the water's buoyancy to make it easier for you to move, or if you just want a change from the routine, these exercises are for you.

As you probably already know, you can stress your back doing everyday tasks, or even by sleeping or sitting in uncomfortable positions. In chapter 5 we help you find the best ways to stand, sit, sleep, drive, work, and do daily chores in order to prevent back pain. A few simple precautions now can save a lot of agony later.

Finally, we provide some sensible recommendations on weight loss and weight management in the last chapter in case you feel that losing weight might lessen the stress on your lower back. We also explain how stress affects back pain and offer a choice of relaxation techniques for those who are experiencing stress (and who isn't).

So start now! If you are one of the millions of people searching for relief from back pain, we'll get you on your way to a better back and a healthier life.

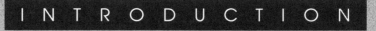

You Are Not Alone

MIKE BACKED HIS TRUCK UP to the loading dock. He was glad this was the last stop of the day. The truck's front end was vibrating terribly and he wanted to get back to the garage to check it out. He cringed as he climbed down from the cab. "I'm getting too old for this," he said and then laughed at himself. He was only 35. He stretched, lit a cigarette, and started unloading bags of cement mix. Hefting the first one went okay, and the second, but as he lifted the third, a familiar pain shot through his lower back. He dropped the bag. . . .

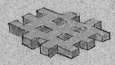

LUISA WAS HAPPY TO BABY-SIT her granddaughter while her daughter was at work. They were in the kitchen together, Connie playing with some old blocks while Luisa made their lunch. Once the table was set, Luisa bent over the block tower and reached for Connie. "Come to Grandma," she said. As she lifted the 3-year-old she felt a snap and a flare of pain in her back. Despite her discomfort, the two had a nice lunch together. But as the afternoon wore on, Luisa's back pain got worse....

TRACY WAS FINISHING HER SHIFT. It had been a busy afternoon—running radar, writing tickets, cruising the expressway, and responding to calls, minor accidents mostly. Traffic was terrible and motorists' tempers were running high. Her back was killing her. She tried to relax, but couldn't. She was anxious to get home so she could pop in a video, kick back, and finish off the last piece of raspberry-chocolate cake....

JAY'S NEW EXECUTIVE POSITION

meant long hours at his desk, countless meetings, and tight deadlines. He thrived on the pressure. Late one evening, as he sifted through computer files and spreadsheets, he casually reached for a file on the shelf behind him. Suddenly his back tightened and began to ache. He tried to ignore the pain. A good workout on the basketball court tomorrow and I'll be fine, he thought. . . .

Do any of these situations sound familiar to you? If not, they may someday, as you have a 7 in 10 chance of experiencing back pain sometime in your adult life.

Back pain is extremely common. It is the major cause of disability in people under 45 and the third cause for people over 45. It is the second most likely cause of absenteeism from work, next to the common cold. And it is one of the most likely reasons for you to see a doctor, especially if that doctor is an orthopedic surgeon, a neurosurgeon, or an osteopath.

Back pain is an equal opportunity condition. It strikes men and women, in blue-collar and white-collar jobs, usually during their most productive work years (their 30s and 40s). In 1990, over 5-1/2 million people lived with disc disorders, and they are only a fraction of those who experience back pain.

Back pain is one of the most costly ailments of working-age adults, although the bulk of the cost is spent on a small number of patients with chronic back pain. The national cost of medical care for back pain in 1984 was over $11.6 billion. Earnings lost because of back pain in that same year reached $2.95 billion. Estimates of money spent on medical care for back pain in 1990 reached over $22.7 billion.

In addition, back pain is a burden on the economy. The total compensable cost for workers' low back pain cases in the U.S. in 1986 was $11.1 billion. This was a 241% increase over 1980's estimated cost of $4.6 billion, a much higher percentage increase than that for all disabilities as a whole during the same time period.

These facts may sound discouraging. But fortunately, the symptoms of up to 90% of those who have back pain decrease over time. And better yet you can take actions to prevent back pain from getting in your way. That's what this book is all about—how you can reduce or avoid back pain.

We hope to show you how minor changes in your lifestyle can make major differences in how you, and your back, feel.

CHAPTER 1

First Aid and Pain Relief for Back Attacks

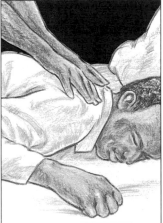

I f you picked up this book because your back hurts, you've come to the right place. Whether your pain is a dull, nagging ache or spasms that incapacitate you, we offer steps you can take immediately to get some relief.

But your first decision should be whether to go to the doctor right now or to wait. Here's some guidance to help you decide what to do.

When Pain First Strikes

Back pain usually is not an emergency medical problem, even when it's very severe. But there are times when back pain may signal serious injury to the nervous system and immediate medical assistance is crucial.

1

See a doctor *immediately* if . . .

- your pain follows an impact injury or some sort of fall or accident.

- your pain follows lifting a heavy object (if you are older).

- you have, in addition to back symptoms, a foot that slaps when you walk or leg muscles that cannot raise you up on your toes.

- you feel, in addition to your back symptoms, continuous tingling, numbness, or weakness in your legs or lower trunk.

- you're running a fever or you have chills and your back symptoms wake you at night but improve when you get up and move around.

- you've lost bowel or bladder control.

Don't delay if you have any one of these symptoms.

See a doctor *soon* if . . .

- you have, in addition to back symptoms, pain that runs down a leg or arm.

- you have swelling or pain in other joints or other parts of the body.

- your pain doesn't improve after a few days' rest and home treatment.

First Aid

If you've decided to treat your backache at home, try these five tips for pain relief.

Stop and Rest

This may seem obvious, but a determined golfer out on the course or an executive with an important project may try to keep going through the pain. Don't! Pain bad enough to limit activity means that your back needs less stress in order to recover. Stop and take a break.

If your pain continues, try getting into a comfortable position. Often that means lying on your back with a small pillow under your knees. Sometimes sitting, or lying on your side with your knees bent, feels better. Another position that often provides relief is lying on your back with your feet resting on a chair. If you do this, be sure to bend your knees 90 degrees and place a rolled towel or small pillow under your neck. Each of these techniques is good for resting the back. Find the position that most relieves your pain and stay there for several hours.

If the pain is very bad, try a day or two of bed rest. Don't stay in bed longer than that unless your doctor prescribes it—too much bed rest can weaken the supporting muscles of the back. Your bed should be very firm; if it isn't, and the pain is severe, try lying on the floor on blankets or other cushioning.

When you rest in bed . . .

- Don't sit up, even though you might want to in order to read or watch TV. Sitting puts more pressure on your spine.

- Get up and move around for 20 to 30 minutes for every 3 hours in bed. Walk slowly or hold on to a counter or sink basin and gently shift your weight from one foot to the other.

- Get into and out of bed carefully. One way to get into bed is to sit on the edge of the left side of the bed if your pain is mostly on your left side (or vice versa). Lower your head and trunk onto your left side and pull your legs up. Then roll gently onto your back. Reverse the sequence to get out of bed, pushing yourself up from the lying position with your arms.

Take a Pain Reliever

Take acetaminophen plus either aspirin or ibuprofen. Don't take aspirin and ibuprofen together, because taking them together won't necessarily increase pain relief and may, in fact, negate their positive effects and increase the likelihood of side effects.

> Do *not* use aspirin or ibuprofen if you have asthma or nasal polyps or are allergic to these medications.

Apply Cold, Then Heat

For the first 48 hours of your pain, use cold to treat your back. Cold will reduce pain, swelling, and muscle spasms.

A simple, safe way to apply cold is to use an ice pack or a plastic bag filled with ice. Apply the bag directly to the skin for 20 minutes at a time. Twenty minutes is plenty of time, don't overdo it! Cold applications can be done three to four times a day.

After 48 hours you might try heat, either instead of or in addition to cold. Heat may relieve pain, but it may also promote swelling and aching after it's been applied. Don't use heat at all if your back pain was caused by an accident, a fall, or a blow to the back.

Apply heat by taking a warm shower or bath or by using a hydrocollator (available at medical supply stores) or a hot water bottle wrapped in a towel. These methods provide moist heat and are safer than heating pads. Apply heat only a couple times a day for 20 minutes at a time.

> Do *not* use cold as a treatment if you have Raynaud's phenomenon or are hypersensitive to cold. Be cautious in using it if you have rheumatoid arthritis.

> To avoid burns,
> - do *not* apply heat to scar tissue, as blood circulation is poor in such tissue and burns easily, and
> - do *not* fall asleep while applying heat.
>
> Heating pads are not recommended.

Get a Gentle Massage

A gentle massage from your spouse or a friend may help stretch and relax tight muscles. Don't try this if your back pain is due to a fall or other injury, and stop immediately if it causes any pain.

Use Relaxation Techniques

Back muscles can contract to protect themselves or other parts of the back. Muscles that are fatigued and overworked may become tense, and then being fatigued by the tension, they may start to hurt. Relaxation can sometimes lessen this pain. We'll discuss relaxation techniques for back pain sufferers later in this book.

Precautions for Life After an Attack

If you follow our first-aid advice, chances are you will gradually feel less pain and begin to get back into your old routine. But you'll want to be careful to not over-work your back as you recover. Try not to bend forward or lift objects, if at all possible, and keep these additional suggestions in mind:

When you sit . . .

- Move around every 20 minutes.

- Use a lower back or foot support if it feels comfortable. For lower or lumbar back supports you can use a rolled-up towel, a small cushion, or a specially made support that can be attached to your chair. Do not use a lower back support if you have been diagnosed as having spondylolisthesis or a kind of spinal stenosis (see chapter 3), as use of the support may aggravate your symptoms.

- Use a chair with armrests, if possible.

- Don't put your legs straight out in front of you.

- Try not to bend or twist as you rise from your seat.

When you drive . . .

- Limit your time in the car when possible.
- Make sure your knees are slightly higher than your hips.
- Use a lower back support if one is not built into your seat.
- Stop frequently to walk around.

If you've tried the home treatments suggested here and if enough time has passed, your back is probably feeling better. But if pain or discomfort persists, you may need to see a physician.

CHAPTER 2

Medical Help for Your Back

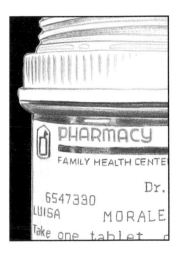

If you're still in pain after following our first-aid suggestions or if you have any of the warning symptoms listed in chapter 1, then you should see a physician. But how do you know which type to see? What questions might the physician ask you? And what are the possible treatments for your condition?

We'll answer all these questions in this chapter, but let's start at the beginning. Who should you see?

Medical Professionals Who Treat Back Pain

If this is your first bout with back pain, you may want to contact a physician who treats the whole body, such as a general practitioner, family physician, or internist, especially if he or she knows you well.

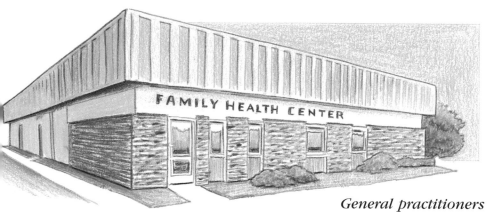

General practitioners are, as their title implies, generalists. They have had medical training and are certified as physicians, but they have not completed residence training for special board certifications.

Family physicians are trained in six basic areas: community medicine, internal medicine, obstetrics and gynecology, pediatrics, surgery, and psychiatry. They have the skills needed for total family care.

Internists deal with the diagnosis and nonsurgical treatment of diseases in adults, except for obstetric problems.

The advantage of going to one of these doctors rather than to a more specialized physician is that they will consider all the possible causes of your back pain. Back pain can be created not only by muscle or bone dysfunctions in the back but also occasionally by a number of other diseases or conditions whose symptoms can seem to be just common back pain. By getting your medical history and doing a physical exam, these doctors can check to make sure one of these ailments is not the cause of your problem.

A disadvantage of seeing these doctors is that they may not have current knowledge of back pain treatment. They may provide passive treatment such as rest or drugs without teaching you how to actively protect your back with exercise or without giving you guidelines about posture, lifting, and bending. If your doctor does not provide information on how to stay active while taking your back into account or if the treatments have not relieved your pain after a few months, you probably need to ask for a referral to a specialist.

Another first choice might be an osteopath. *Osteopaths* are trained much like other physicians, though through a different system, and are licensed to practice medicine. They have an additional focus on the treatment of muscles, bones, and joints. Osteopaths believe that musculoskeletal system imbalances and abnormalities may affect the proper functioning of the musculoskeletal system and other body systems. They may use their hands to manipulate the musculoskeletal system as part of treatment.

Physician specialists that you may be referred to include these:

Orthopedic surgeons specialize in the treatment of bones and joints. They perform surgery, care for fractures, and treat diseases of the bones and joints. As well as using casts and braces, orthopedic surgeons may also prescribe excrcises and supervise physical therapy. They are often consulted for back problems.

Physiatrists design physical therapy and rehabilitation programs to help patients function better in daily life. They choose exercises and other forms of treatment to relieve pain and promote easier movement. Physiatrists instruct the physical therapists who administer therapy, and they monitor patients' progress. This specialist has a wide range of types of treatment to offer.

Neurosurgeons focus on the brain, spinal cord, and peripheral nerves of the body. They often deal with injuries to the brain or spinal cord resulting from trauma or tumors.

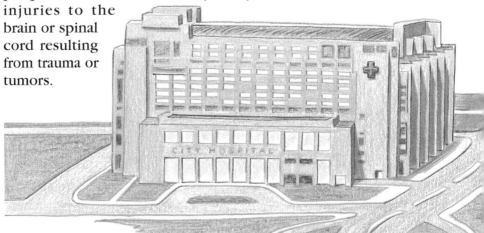

Three other health care professionals you may work with are the physical therapist, the kinesiotherapist, and the occupational therapist. All require a bachelor's or master's degree. They work under a physician's direction and with other health care personnel as part of a team.

Physical therapists work with patients to carry out exercise regimens. They keep track of individual progress and adjust treatment as necessary. In addition to exercise, they may use massage, heat, cold, light, water, and electrical stimulation to try to reduce symptoms. They may also teach patients how to carry out treatment at home.

Kinesiotherapists do much the same work as physical therapists, but they tend to specialize in therapeutic exercise, physical fitness, and patient education for those needing rehabilitation, especially long-term.

Occupational therapists evaluate, diagnose, and treat people with physical or mental impairments. They focus on helping people develop or restore their ability to carry out daily tasks at home or at work. This may include teaching patients how to use mechanical aids that extend their ability to function, such as splints and crutches.

Another type of health care professional you may choose to see is a chiropractor.

Chiropractors are health practitioners, but they go through different training and licensing than physicians. They attend special 4-year chiropractic colleges that emphasize spinal adjustment and study of nerves, muscles, joints, posture, exercise, and nutrition.

Chiropractors focus on the proper functioning of the spine and nervous system. Much of their work relates to back pain. One of their primary forms of treatment is manipulation—the use of the hands to apply force to parts of the spine in order to adjust the spine. They may use therapies similar to those of physical therapists (heat and cold, massage, water therapy); they also may recommend rest, exercise, diet, and the use of braces or other supports for the back or other parts of the body. Chiropractors may not prescribe prescription drugs or perform surgery.

Chiropractic treatment is somewhat controversial. Some chiropractors claim that chiropractic treatment can cure medical problems beyond those directly related to muscle or bone alignment, yet many physicians do not believe that manipulation of the spine is an effective treatment for any medical problem. Manipulation does relieve pain for some patients, although sometimes only on a short-term basis. It also carries some risk; in rare cases, permanent injury has resulted from manipulation.

Once you have decided whom to see, you need to prepare for your first consultation. Your doctor makes decisions based on the information you provide, so the more accurately you can describe your problem, the more effectively your doctor can treat you.

Preparing to See the Doctor

Doctors are a bit like detectives—they are trained to search for clues that point to a specific cause for your back pain, which is often difficult or even impossible to determine. They also look for clues that, along with their training and experience, help them choose appropriate care for your particular case.

Before you visit your doctor, think about the following questions and how they apply to you.

DR. CARMEN MENDEZ

Back Pain Clues

1. Have you had back pain before? If so, when?

2. When did your current back pain start? What do you think triggered it?

3. What types of symptoms do you have—pain, numbness, weakness, stiffness?

4. Where is the pain located? Is it just in the back or just in the neck? Does it radiate to other parts of the body? Is it constant, or is it intermittent?

5. Are some positions—for example, sitting, standing, or lying down—more comfortable than others? What, if anything, makes the pain worse? Better?

6. Is the pain getting worse or better? Are attacks becoming more frequent or less frequent?

7. Have the symptoms changed since they began? How?

8. How do your symptoms interfere with what you do in daily life?

9. What tests have previously been done on your spine, and what were the results? (If the doctor you are going to see does not have these results on record, have them sent or take them with you.)

10. What treatments have you tried in the past? How effective were they?

11. Have you had other diseases, operations, or joint problems?

12. Does your job stress you emotionally or require manual labor?

13. Do you stand a lot in your job? Sit? Drive?

14. Do you get any regular exercise?

15. Are there other stressors in your life? How do you usually handle stress?

16. What kinds of back problems have other family members had?

If there are points you feel are significant about your condition that your doctor doesn't bring up, be sure to mention them. This will help you and your doctor better understand the problem and, if you have lengthy medical records, this will ensure that the doctor hasn't missed any pertinent medical history.

Common Treatments for Back Pain

Once your doctor has examined you, he or she will prescribe treatment. A wide range of possibilities is available, so we'll acquaint you with the most common ones. If you're not sure about some of the anatomical terms mentioned in this section, check in chapter 3, where the parts of the spine are described.

Rest

As we suggested you do in the last chapter, resting by lying in bed or otherwise restricting movement is probably the most common, and safest, thing to do for back pain. It relieves the pain and aids recovery.

Drugs

Four types of drugs may be prescribed for back pain: analgesics, muscle relaxants, anti-inflammatories, and, for extreme pain, narcotics.

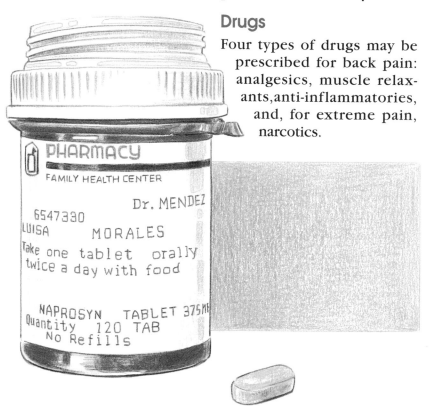

PHARMACY
FAMILY HEALTH CENTER
Dr. MENDEZ
6547330
LUISA   MORALES
Take one tablet   orally
twice a day with food

NAPROSYN   TABLET 375MG
Quantity   120 TAB
No Refills

Drugs Commonly Prescribed for Back Pain

Type	Action	Recommendation for use
Analgesics (acetaminophen)	Reduce pain	To be used for mild to moderate pain. Safe for long-term use. Avoid stomach upset sometimes caused by anti-inflammatory drugs. Can be used in combination with other drugs.
Anti-inflammatory drugs (aspirin, ibuprofen, Indocin, Motrin, Naprosyn, Butazolidin)	Reduce swelling, inflammation; some reduce pain	To reduce inflammation and pain. Most are safe for long-term use. Some side effects are possible, such as stomach discomfort. Butazolidin and Indocin can have serious side effects.
Muscle relaxants (Valium, carisoprodol, diazepam)	Depress the nervous system to tranquilize the body	To relax muscles in spasm. No clear advantage over non-steroidal anti-inflammatories. Short-term use only. Can act as mood depressants. Addictive potential. Depress the body's own endorphins.
Narcotic drugs (morphine, codeine, Demerol, Percodan, Darvon, Talwin)	Depress the nervous system to relieve pain	To be used only for extreme pain. Addictive potential. Short-term use only. Many side effects. Depress the body's own endorphins.

In addition to these drugs, injections of anesthetic solutions, with or without corticosteroids, may be made into facet joints (joints that interlock around the vertebrae and help keep the vertebrae aligned) or into the space around the spinal nerves. Such injections may carry some risk of complications. Also, some recent studies have brought into question the effectiveness of these injections.

Physical Therapy and Exercise

Physical therapists have a number of pain- and spasm-relieving treatments for back pain:

- Heat or cold, applied in the form of hot or cold packs, cryotherapy machines, ultrasound, or hot and cold whirlpool baths

- Massage

- TENS, or transcutaneous electrical nerve stimulation, passes a small electrical current through the skin using electrodes (the efficacy of this treatment has been questioned)

- Passive mobilization or movement of specific spinal segments

Most physical therapists will also teach patients with back pain a set of exercises to practice on a daily basis. Some therapists use biofeedback—electronic monitoring that helps patients see or hear how effectively they are performing exercises.

Mechanical Spinal Supports

Some type of spinal support, like a corset, backbrace, or elasticized undergarment, is sometimes prescribed. These are meant to give support to and reduce mechanical stress on the lower spine. Occasionally they are used to help support the abdomen in overweight patients or just after surgery to protect the weakened back from stress.

The disadvantage of such supports is that over time they may reduce the conditioning of the trunk muscles. Back muscles and tendons may stiffen, and the wearer may develop a psychological dependence on the support as a means to avoid pain. Because back pain may be caused or worsened by weak muscles, it's best not to wear a support longer than is necessary. In fact, no studies have proven the efficacy of mechanical supports. If your doctor does prescribe one, you should talk to him or her about conditioning exercises to counteract any muscle deconditioning that might occur.

Traction

Traction is the application of a stretching force to the spine by means of either an attached weight or gravity against one's own body weight. It can be done while the patient lies in bed or while he or she is strapped into a special upright apparatus. Traction is applied several times a day for a number of weeks or months.

The idea behind traction is to separate the vertebrae to remove pressure from damaged discs and possibly allow more nutrients to diffuse into the discs. It has not been proven to be effective, and there is growing evidence that it is not useful for those who have disc herniations or sciatica (pain that runs down the legs).

Surgery

Surgery is a good choice for only a very small number of back problems. It is often not successful. For example, out of all patients who undergo disc removal to control sciatica, only 60% achieve complete relief.

More conservative measures should be tried before surgery unless there is some imminent risk of neurological damage.

If surgery is recommended for your back problem, learn as much as you can from your doctor or other reputable medical sources about the procedure. Ask questions about the purpose of the surgery, what will be done during the operation, and what risks are involved. Find out how the surgery may affect your body, both immediately following the operation and after healing has taken place, and whether additional treatment or restrictions will be necessary following surgery. If possible, get a second opinion before having surgery.

Whatever the treatment your doctor prescribes, talk with him or her about its purpose and potential outcomes. As treatment ensues, let your doctor know how you think you're doing in relation to the desired outcomes. Keeping those lines of communication open will help your doctor effectively evaluate your treatment and adjust it if necessary.

By reading this far, we hope you've learned about a home treatment or medical treatment that will help relieve your back pain. But there's more to learn, and more you can do. By understanding how the back works, what can go wrong, and what the controllable risk factors are, you can make lifestyle choices that will help you avoid future back pain.

CHAPTER 3

How Your Back Works and Why It Sometimes Doesn't

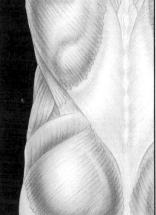

T he fact is, a lot of how we function every day is due to the hard work and support of our back and spine. Not only does the spine protect the spinal cord, from which most nerves originate, but it also supports the body and allows us to turn and bend right or left, backward or forward, with great freedom of motion. The many muscles that attach to and reinforce the spine connect with other parts of the body to allow movement.

The spine is the center of an elaborate web of nerves, bones, and muscles meant to work together to keep us upright, moving, and sensing what goes on around us. Given the spine's complexity and the amount of force we place on it (hundreds of pounds of force in the course of a normal day), it may be more surprising that something *doesn't* go wrong more often.

21

Let's take a guided tour of the back and examine some of its main components.

The Structure of the Spine

The spine is a stack of 26 bones, called *vertebrae* (the plural form of *vertebra*), alternating with pads of soft tissue, called *discs*. This stack is held together by ligaments that run both between separate vertebrae and along the entire spine. The back muscles attach to projections on the vertebrae.

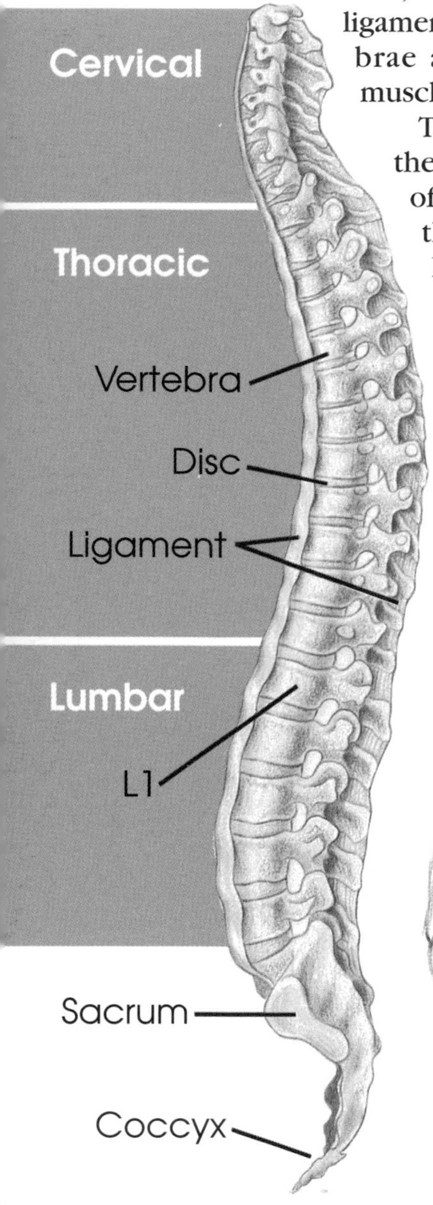

The entire spine is essentially made up of the same materials, although different areas of the spine connect with different parts of the body and have specialized functions. For ease of identification, the vertebrae are labeled using a sequential letter and number system. The letter is taken from the name of the region that each vertebra resides in, and the number is taken from the vertebra's position in that region, top to bottom. For example, L1 would be the first vertebra in the lumbar region.

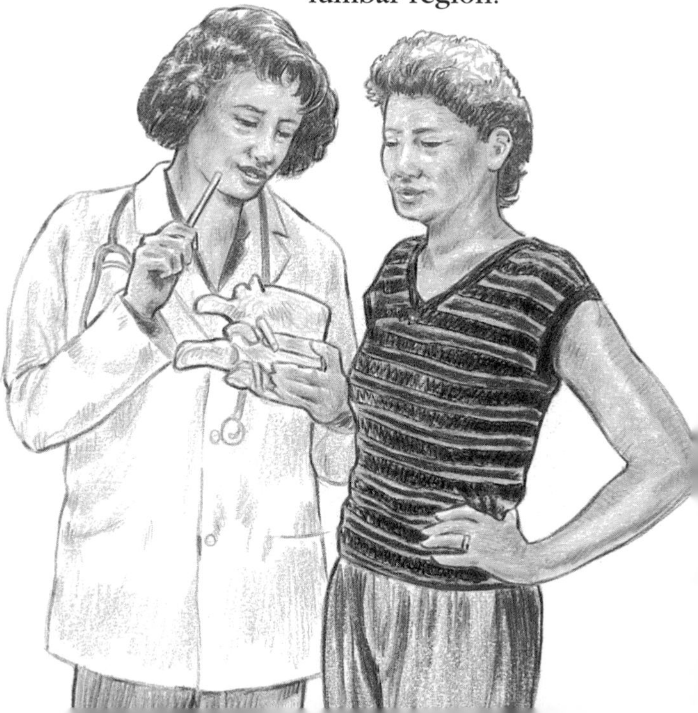

Cervical

Thoracic

Vertebra

Disc

Ligament

Lumbar

L1

Sacrum

Coccyx

Now let's go in for a closer look at the vertebrae and discs.

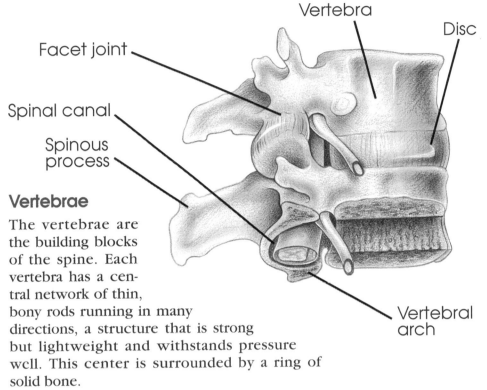

Vertebra

Disc

Facet joint

Spinal canal

Spinous process

Vertebral arch

Vertebrae

The vertebrae are the building blocks of the spine. Each vertebra has a central network of thin, bony rods running in many directions, a structure that is strong but lightweight and withstands pressure well. This center is surrounded by a ring of solid bone.

An arch is also formed on the back of each vertebra. If you put your hand on your back, you can feel the ridgelike tops of those arches, called the *spinous processes*. To either side of them are the *facet joints*, which interlock and serve as a guidance system for keeping the vertebrae properly aligned.

Besides supporting the back, the vertebrae protect the spinal cord from damage. The *vertebral arches* form the *spinal canal*, through which the spinal cord passes. Nerves branch from the spinal cord between the vertebrae to extend to other parts of the body. When you realize that nerves pass through the vertebrae, it becomes easier to understand how protruding disc material or a shift in a vertebra can cause pain, both in the back and in other parts of the body.

Endplate

Nucleus
pulposus

Anulus
fibrosus

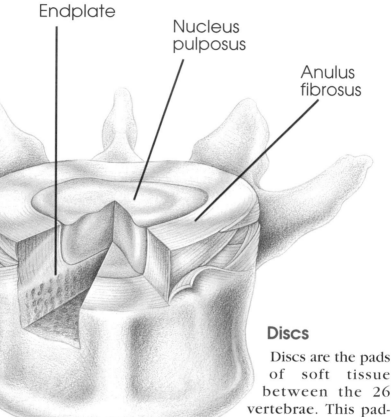

Discs

Discs are the pads
of soft tissue
between the 26
vertebrae. This pad-
ding allows the bony
spine to twist more easily. Discs
have a gel-like center, called the *nucleus pulposus*, surrounded by a layered ring of fibrous tissue, called the
anulus fibrosus. The anulus absorbs most of the load
when the spine is jarred, but the nucleus helps distrib-
ute that load evenly.

Above and below each disc are layers of connective
tissue called *endplates*. Through early childhood,
blood vessels penetrate the endplates and carry nutrients directly to the disc, but this gradually changes as
we grow. By adolescence, discs no longer have their
own blood supply. Blood vessels from the vertebrae
only touch the endplates, indirectly providing nutrients to the rest of the disc.

The Ligaments and Muscles of the Back

The vertebrae and discs of the spine provide a basic structure, but flexible connections are needed to keep the bony parts together. And it would be impossible to turn, bend, and move without the muscles of the back to assist us.

Ligaments, the tissues that connect bones to bones, hold the spine together. These bundles of strong, tough fibers bind the vertebrae, keeping them in place.

However, ligaments aren't strong enough to do the job alone when we move, lift, or turn. That's when groups of muscles come into play; the work to be performed dictates which muscle groups will be used.

Hip and leg muscles as well as back muscles are involved when you lift a heavy weight. Back muscles alone are used for lighter work, and your abdominal muscles assist as needed. It's especially important that the muscles be strong enough to sustain whatever effort you put forth; otherwise the ligaments may have to withstand the force alone.

These muscle groups spread the load on the spine more evenly and provide support, preventing injury to the spine. This self-regulating system is effective most of the time, but it can be defeated by sudden movements or overloading, especially when the muscles are weakened and fatigued.

Now you know something about how the back should work. But, since you're reading this book, chances are something went wrong. Here are some of the ways this system can fail.

Possible Causes of Back Pain

Back pain can be created by diseases, congenital defects, and infections as well as by mechanical problems with the spine. Even when the problem can be traced to the spine, it's usually difficult for doctors to pinpoint the specific cause.

A few likely culprits are problems related to back muscles, discs, and facet joints. We'll start with these, then consider some other possibilities.

Muscle Spasms or Injury

Back pain is most likely to occur when our muscles are not up to the task of protecting the back. This can happen when they are not conditioned because we aren't active enough, when they are fatigued, or when we subject them to sudden forces or heavy loads.

Muscle spasm usually signals irritation, though rarely do we know which part of the back is irritated. Fortunately, most of the time relief can be found from rest, ice, and over-the-counter pain relievers.

Muscle spasms may be related to muscle strain or ligament sprain because spasms, like strains and sprains, commonly occur with sudden movement or with prolonged stretching of the back. However, most back symptoms subside faster than those of strains or sprains in other parts of the body; few require a long recovery time.

Disc Bulging and Tearing

By the time we're teens, our discs no longer have direct blood flow, so they gradually become drier and more fibrous. Over time, the nucleus loses water and is less able to sustain pressure. This forces the surrounding anulus to support more of the load.

As aging continues, small tears may form in the anulus, allowing the nucleus to bulge a bit. This bulging is not usually accompanied by pain. However, if the tears increase in size or number the nucleus may leak out and inflame or impinge on an adjacent nerve. This herniation can result in back pain as well as pain in other parts of the body. Such pain felt in the hip or leg is often called sciatica; disorders other than a herniated disc can also cause it.

By the way, there is no such thing as a "slipped" disc. The discs are well connected to the rest of the spine by fibers and ligaments. The term herniated disc is a more accurate description.

Besides the pain that may be caused by damage to the disc itself, disc shrinkage due to deterioration may adversely affect how the facet joints above and below it interact.

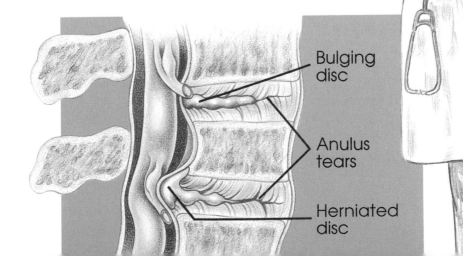

Bulging disc

Anulus tears

Herniated disc

Facet Joint Changes

Facet joints are joints, just like your knee is a joint. Each one is encapsulated with a sac of fluid that lubricates it. Facet joints guide motion in the back and share the load with the discs.

Pressure, often due to changes in a disc, can cause changes to the facet joints, changes that might be capable of causing pain. In severe cases, as can happen in the elderly, facet joint changes can also allow shifting of the vertebrae.

We've covered three of the possible causes of back pain. Here are some additional ones.

Spondylolisthesis

Spondylolisthesis is the slipping forward of part or all of a vertebra onto another. In the lower back this results from stress fractures, defects in the vertebra, or a degenerative disc that allows the vertebra to slide. If the slipped vertebra distorts or presses on a nerve, it can cause back pain or sciatica. In the neck, possible causes are injury, rheumatoid arthritis, or congenital defects. Here spondylolisthesis can create pain and stiffness in the neck and, in severe cases, pain, numbness, or weakness in the hands and arms.

Central Spinal Stenosis

In central spinal stenosis, the spinal canal has become too small for the nerves and spinal cord. Although the canal can be congenitally smaller than normal, it is enlargement or movement of a disc or a vertebra that narrows the canal enough to cause pain. These changes usually come with aging. Bony enlargements often develop around discs and facet joints, and ligaments may fold, diminishing the space in the spinal canal for nerves. The pain from central spinal stenosis often appears in the legs rather than in the back. Numbness or strange sensations such as coldness or rubberiness may develop in the legs.

Damaged Vertebrae Due to Osteoporosis

Throughout our lives, our bones go through a continuous process of being built up, then reabsorbed into the bloodstream. Our bones are thickest when we are young adults; after that, the mechanism that builds bone slows down, due to aging and a reduction in activity, and we gradually lose bone mass. If we grow up with bones that have sufficient mass, that loss is less likely to be significant; but if we begin with less bone mass or if we have rapid bone loss, it's possible to lose so much mass that the bones become brittle and, no longer able to withstand the forces of daily living, are easily crushed. This condition is called osteoporosis.

In osteoporosis, the inner structure of bone, which in strong bone is a tight, thick net, begins to thin, weaken, and become more porous. Like all bones, the vertebrae can be damaged by osteoporosis. Vertebrae are more likely to crush than to break. If this happens, the pain may not occur immediately, but may develop hours after the vertebra has been crushed instead.

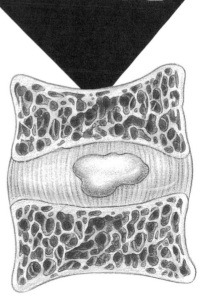

Osteoporosis is more common in older women than in older men for two reasons:

1. Women start out with less bone mass than men.

2. The hormone estrogen facilitates the bone-building process and the absorption of calcium, so there is a rapid drop in bone mass after menopause, when the woman's body produces less estrogen.

Because it is easier to prevent osteoporosis than it is to treat it, John F. Aloia, MD, author of *Osteoporosis: A Guide to Prevention and Treatment*, suggests you follow these guidelines.

Recommendations for Preventing Osteoporosis

1. Get enough calcium in a balanced diet.

2. Get enough vitamin D in your diet and from sunshine.

3. Limit your intake of caffeine, salt, protein, and phosphorus.

4. Do not go on excessively low-calorie diets.

5. Exercise regularly.

6. Take estrogen or progesterone after menopause.

7. Take estrogen if your ovaries have been surgically removed.

8. Avoid drugs that decrease bone mass.

9. Drink alcohol only in moderation.

10. Do not smoke.

Pregnancy

Many studies have shown that half of all pregnant women have back pain during their pregnancy. Pregnancy brings many changes to women's bodies, and the back is one area likely to be affected. Three factors may be involved.

First, the growing baby pushes out the mother's abdomen, moving her center of gravity forward. As the abdominal muscles are stretched, the lower back muscles are stressed.

Second, in the latter half of pregnancy, fibrous structures in the lower back and pelvis soften due to hormonal changes. This allows increased stretching of ligaments.

Third, the outer rings of the discs in the lower back soften, making them more vulnerable to damage, especially if previously injured.

Controllable Risk Factors

Luckily for us, there are a number of factors that we can control to reduce the likelihood of back pain. To see how much at risk you are, take this quiz to find out how many of these factors apply to you.

Self-Quiz

1. _____ Am I overweight?

2. _____ Does my stomach stick out?

3. _____ Do I smoke, especially heavily?

4. _____ Does my work require a lot of sitting, especially without breaks?

5. _____ Is my chair at work comfortable?

6. _____ Does my work entail repetitive pushing and pulling movements or lifting while bending or twisting? (This applies whether you're working at home, in an office, in a warehouse, or outdoors.)

7. _____ Does my work require me to use power tools or heavy moving equipment or to drive a lot?

8. _____ Is my bed comfortable?

9. _____ Do I stand in one place a lot when I work, at home or on the job?

10. _____ Do I slouch most of the time?

11. _____ Is my car seat comfortable for me?

12. _____ Do I engage in any kind of exercise or sport regularly?

13. _____ Does stress in my daily life make my back pain worse?

14. _____ Do I get enough calcium in my diet, especially if I'm over 50?

Now that you've checked your own personal risk factors, let's talk more about what each factor is and how to change it.

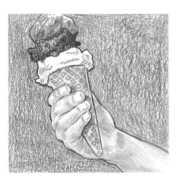

Overweight (Items 1 and 2)

If you're overweight, you probably aren't physically fit, and fitness has been shown to be related to back health. If some of that weight is a potbelly, it may be additionally stressing your lower back muscles.

Our back protection plan includes regular exercise (chapter 4) and weight management (chapter 6).

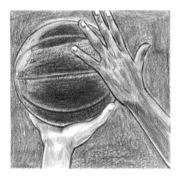

Risky Movements
(Items 6, 7, 11, and 12)

Whether you're on the job, at home, or playing sports, there are certain movements that increase stress on your spine. Lifting is one; lifting as you bend or twist is even worse. Repetitive back movements, such as pitching a softball or working on an assembly line, can also tire muscles and cause pain. Vibration from machinery (a car, a jackhammer) is another culprit.

Knowing the correct posture for lifting, driving, and other work and household tasks can afford you some protection. See chapter 5 for this information.

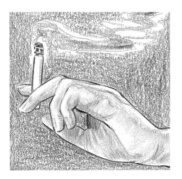

Smoking (Item 3)

The connection between smoking and back pain is not obvious, but a number of studies have shown a strong relationship between the two. Researchers still aren't sure what the connection is. Some speculate that smoking causes coughing, which in turn stresses back muscles. Recent studies indicate that smoking accelerates aging by reducing the blood flow around the discs, depriving them of nutrients.

We won't tackle the struggle of quitting smoking in this book, but because smoking puts you at risk for cancer, heart disease, and many other serious illnesses, as well as for back pain, we suggest you quit if you now smoke.

Being Sedentary
(Items 4 and 12)

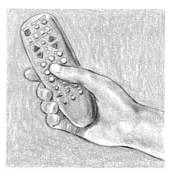

Studies have shown that those who are most fit are the ones least likely to have back pain (not counting sports injuries). This probably is in part because the muscles that support your back are conditioned by exercise; regular aerobic exercise may also more directly help the discs in the back by increasing the blood flow around them, supplying more nutrients. In addition, weight-bearing exercise (such as walking or jogging) helps maintain or increase your bone mass, which helps prevent osteoporosis.

Besides getting regular aerobic exercise, you can improve the strength and flexibility of the muscles that support your back with exercises that focus on those particular muscles. These aren't located only in your back—your abdominal and leg muscles play a large part as well.

In chapter 4, we'll present ideas on how you can get started in an exercise program that will benefit your back—and the rest of you.

Bad Posture (Items 4, 5, 8–11)

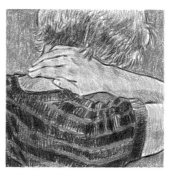

Slouching or slumping won't necessarily do permanent damage to your back, but it can cause pain. Like the other muscles in your body, those in your neck and back can become fatigued if held in one position too long, especially if they have to be tensed to support your body weight.

The obvious solution is to sit and stand in ways that relieve stress on muscles and to move and stretch more often. Having a comfortable bed and chair can help ease back pain as well. We'll give you some hints for daily living in chapter 5.

Pain and Stress (Item 13)

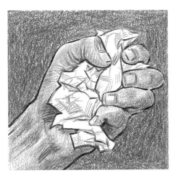

Back pain, like any pain, is likely to feel worse when you're under stress. Conscious relaxation may help you reduce your pain by relaxing tense muscles and lowering your stress level.

We'll offer you some stress-relieving techniques in chapter 6.

Lack of Calcium (Item 14)

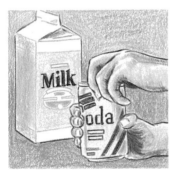

As we mentioned earlier, an adequate supply of calcium throughout your life can provide some protection against developing osteoporosis in old age. You don't have to drink milk if you hate it; other foods can supply calcium, or you can ask your doctor about calcium supplements.

Learn more about how to improve your calcium intake in chapter 6, where you'll also learn some basics of good nutrition.

Now that you're aware of how your back works and what risk factors you can control, it's time to start taking action. One of the best moves you can make to help both your back and your general health is to exercise.

CHAPTER 4

Getting Your Back on Track With Exercise

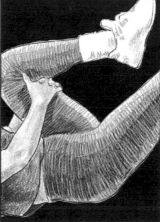

Once the acute pain of your first back attack is over, you'll feel relieved and want to put the whole thing behind you. Unfortunately, one of the best predictors of future back pain is prior back pain. Back symptoms tend to recur.

To help prevent recurrence, you need to condition your back-supporting muscles. We've got three levels of exercises for you to try, starting with very gentle ones and progressing to more vigorous ones. Make these part of your daily routine: A 20-minute workout may save you days of pain. Or use them in conjunction with your favorite type of aerobic exercise, one that keeps you moving continuously and makes you sweat. Studies have shown that fitness correlates with less back pain.

Exercise is *not* a panacea for all back pain. Before you begin, here are a few words of caution.

The exercises in this chapter are not appropriate if your pain

- is unremitting, regardless of your posture,
- is the result of a traumatic accident,
- involves bowel or bladder problems,
- follows an illness or fever,
- is severe and extends below the knee, or
- includes numbness, weakness, or tingling below the knee.

If your pain is like any of these, get professional guidance before beginning an exercise program. Although some of these symptoms can result from mechanical dysfunctions of the spine, it is possible that they are being generated by other conditions unrelated to the spine. An exercise good for one person will not necessarily work for the person whose symptoms are from a different cause. This means you must use common sense.

If an exercise hurts you, *stop doing it*! It may not be appropriate for your condition, or you may be performing it incorrectly. In either case, you need a medical professional to advise you before you try it again.

If pain or discomfort persists when you try a specific exercise, especially after you've asked for advice on your exercise performance, drop the part of the exercise that hurts. For example, if you are performing an exercise that involves bending forward or bending backward and the pain occurs only in the last few degrees of movement, stop prior to the point where it begins to hurt. You may find that after you've done this for a few days, the discomfort may subside, and you may be able to do the entire exercise. However, if the pain does not subside, continue leaving out the part that causes it.

A few more points to remember:

- If you are presently experiencing severe to moderate pain, you probably should wait until your symptoms lessen before beginning this exercise program.

- Seek professional medical advice before starting this or any other exercise program.

- If any exercise causes leg pain or tingling, discontinue it.

- If you have osteoporosis, be careful when doing exercises that flex the back, that is, that make you bend forward.

- For movements that are held for several seconds, start by holding for a length of time that does not cause pain, even if that is less than the recommended amount. As your muscles become stronger and more flexible, gradually increase the amount of time you hold each position until you reach the recommended maximum.

- Perform each exercise in a slow, controlled fashion. Never move jerkily or quickly. Sudden movements can cause minor injury, and they do not promote flexibility as well as slower ones do.

- Don't force any movement beyond where you feel comfortable. Everyone's body differs in its normal alignment, so don't push it beyond where it seems right. *This is especially important for your back.*

Before you exercise, warm up your body by walking or riding a stationary bike for 5 to 10 minutes at an easy pace. This will warm your muscles slightly, making it easier to stretch.

When you exercise, do it in a quiet room, with no distractions. It's best to exercise on a carpeted floor to cushion your back; an exercise mat can be used on an uncarpeted floor. Wear loose-fitting clothing that won't restrict your motion.

As you perform each exercise, breathe normally. (In some exercises we have noted natural places to inhale or exhale.) Don't hold your breath as you move. Keep your movements slow and controlled, especially when performing a number of repetitions.

Start with the Level 1 exercises presented here. When you've mastered most of the exercises at Level 1, move to Level 2. Finally, when you are able to perform most of the exercises at Level 2 at the maximum repetitions, go to Level 3.

Level 1

Level 1 is appropriate for those just starting an exercise program. Even if you think you are fairly fit, you should at least practice and become familiar with these exercises, because Levels 2 and 3 build on Level 1.

PELVIC TILT (STANDING)

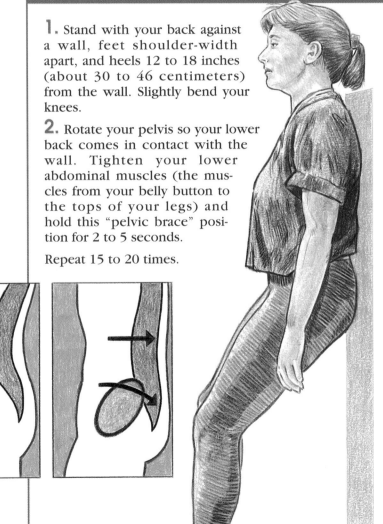

1. Stand with your back against a wall, feet shoulder-width apart, and heels 12 to 18 inches (about 30 to 46 centimeters) from the wall. Slightly bend your knees.

2. Rotate your pelvis so your lower back comes in contact with the wall. Tighten your lower abdominal muscles (the muscles from your belly button to the tops of your legs) and hold this "pelvic brace" position for 2 to 5 seconds.

Repeat 15 to 20 times.

PELVIC TILT
(ON YOUR BACK)

1. Lie on your back with both knees bent, feet flat on the floor, and arms at your sides. (You may wish to place a small pillow under your head or neck.)

2. Exhale and rotate your pelvis so your lower back comes in contact with the floor. Tighten your lower abdominal muscles and hold this "pelvic brace" position for 2 to 5 seconds.

Repeat 15 to 20 times.

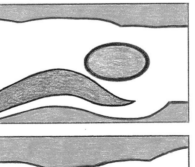

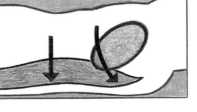

BACK ARCH

1. Get on all fours on the floor and pull in your abdominal muscles.

2. Drop your head forward and round your back as you tilt your pelvis. Hold for 5 seconds. (See the pelvic tilt exercises if you have trouble understanding how to tilt your pelvis.)

Repeat 5 to 10 times.

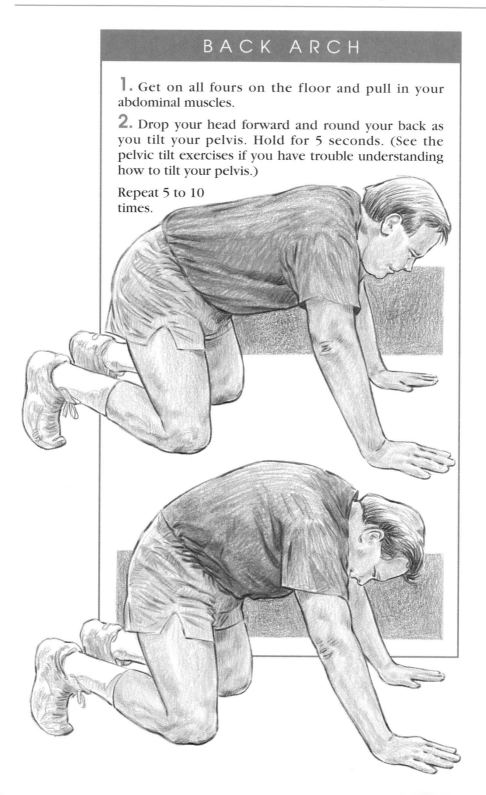

KNEES TO CHEST

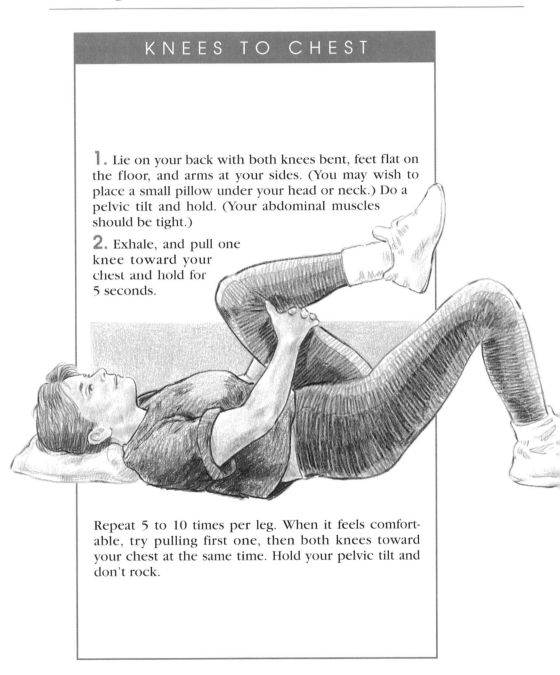

1. Lie on your back with both knees bent, feet flat on the floor, and arms at your sides. (You may wish to place a small pillow under your head or neck.) Do a pelvic tilt and hold. (Your abdominal muscles should be tight.)

2. Exhale, and pull one knee toward your chest and hold for 5 seconds.

Repeat 5 to 10 times per leg. When it feels comfortable, try pulling first one, then both knees toward your chest at the same time. Hold your pelvic tilt and don't rock.

LEG RAISE

1. Lie on your back with both knees bent, feet flat on the floor, and arms at your sides. (You may wish to place a small pillow under your head or neck.) Do a pelvic tilt and hold. (Your abdominal muscles should be tight.)

2. Exhale, and straighten one knee and slowly raise your leg as high as possible without pain. (Do not allow your pelvis to rock or to roll upward.) Try to keep your leg straight without locking your knee. Hold this position for 5 seconds, then slowly return it to the floor.

Repeat 5 to 10 times per leg.

PRONE ON ELBOWS

1. Lie facedown on the floor with your arms at your sides and your head turned to one side. Take deep breaths and try to relax for 3 to 5 minutes.

2. Place your elbows under your shoulders as you ease your trunk up, then rest your weight on your forearms. (Use your shoulders and arms to push your head and upper trunk up; do *not* use your back muscles to lift.) Look straight ahead. Hold this position for 15 to 30 seconds.

Do once per exercise session.

Level 2

Move to exercises from this level only when you are able to do most of the Level 1 exercises for the maximum number of repetitions and hold the movement for the maximum number of seconds *for a few days in a row.* How well you can perform an exercise may vary from day to day, so wait until you can consistently meet the maximums.

WALL SLIDE

1. Stand with your back against a wall, feet shoulder-width apart, and heels 12 to 18 inches (about 30 to 46 centimeters) from the wall. Slightly bend your knees.

2. Exhale, and rotate your pelvis so your lower back comes in contact with the wall. Tighten your lower abdominal muscles and hold.

3. Bend your knees while sliding your back down the wall. Initially just bend your knees slightly; when you are comfortable with that, go a bit farther and then a bit farther. Do not ever bend your knees more than 90 degrees. Hold the bottom position for 10 to 20 seconds.

Repeat 5 to 10 times. This exercise also strengthens your abdominal and thigh muscles. Try to build up to holding for 2 minutes. If your knees hurt, try bending them only slightly. Reduce the number of repetitions as you increase the length for which you hold each repetition.

QUADRUPED

1. Get on all fours on the floor. Brace your pelvis by pulling in your abdominals and holding your back in a pain-free position.

2. Slowly raise each arm and each leg, one at a time, to a horizontal position. Hold each up for 5 seconds, then lower it. Do not allow your trunk to sag by maintaining your pelvic brace, and keep your eyes on the floor.

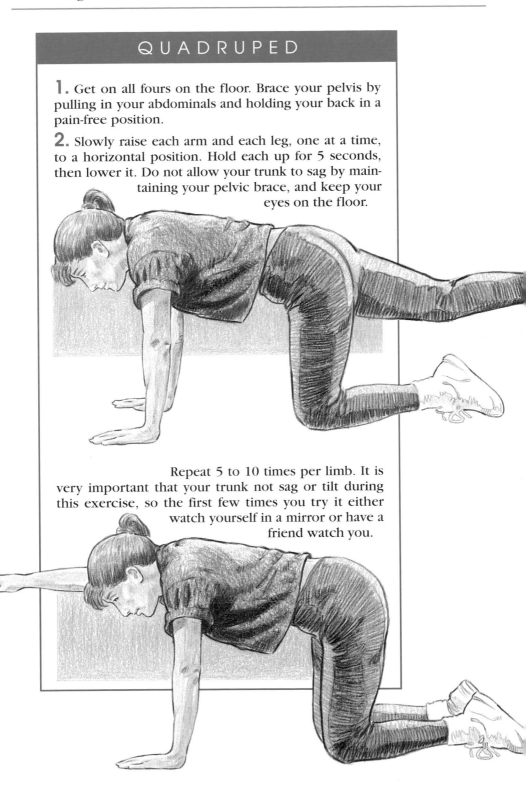

Repeat 5 to 10 times per limb. It is very important that your trunk not sag or tilt during this exercise, so the first few times you try it either watch yourself in a mirror or have a friend watch you.

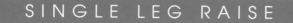

SINGLE LEG RAISE

1. Lie on your back with both knees bent, feet flat on the floor, and arms at your sides. (You may wish to place a small pillow under your head or neck.) Exhale, do a pelvic tilt, and hold.

2. Straighten one knee and slowly raise your leg as high as possible without pain. (Do not point or flex your foot.) After you have raised your leg as far as you can, keeping your knee straight but not locked, gently pull your leg closer to you as you contract the front of your thigh. Hold for 10 seconds.

Repeat 5 to 10 times per leg. Your goal should be to raise each leg a minimum of 80 degrees off the floor.

If you have sciatica, consult with your physician before attempting the Single Leg Raise. Don't do it when your sciatica is painful.

HIP FLEXOR STRETCH

1. Lie on your back with legs straight and arms at your sides.

2. Grasp one thigh behind your knee and pull it toward your chest until your lower back is in contact with the floor. Keep the opposite leg straight at the same time.

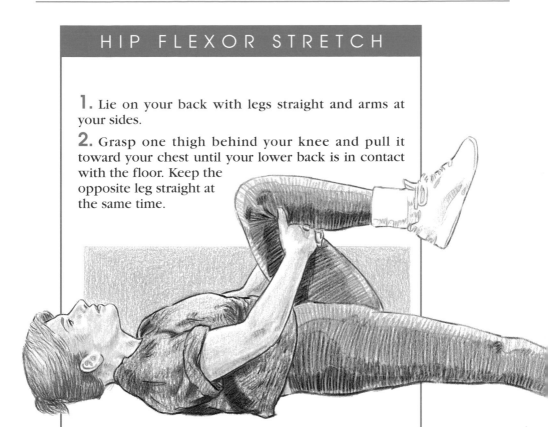

3. If your extended leg does not stay on the floor, hold this position 5 to 10 seconds. If you are doing this exercise correctly and your extended leg *is* in contact with the floor, you don't need to perform this exercise.

Repeat 5 to 10 times per leg if your extended leg does not stay on the floor. If it does, eliminate this exercise from your routine; however, you may want to try this exercise periodically to make sure your hip flexors are still flexible.

TRUNK CURL

1. Lie on your back with both knees bent and feet flat on the floor. Cross your arms across your chest, do a pelvic tilt, and hold.

2. Keeping your lower back in contact with the floor, exhale and slowly raise your shoulder blades off the floor, then lower them, inhaling as you return to the starting position. Keep your eyes on the ceiling; try not to bend your neck forward.

Repeat 15 to 30 times.

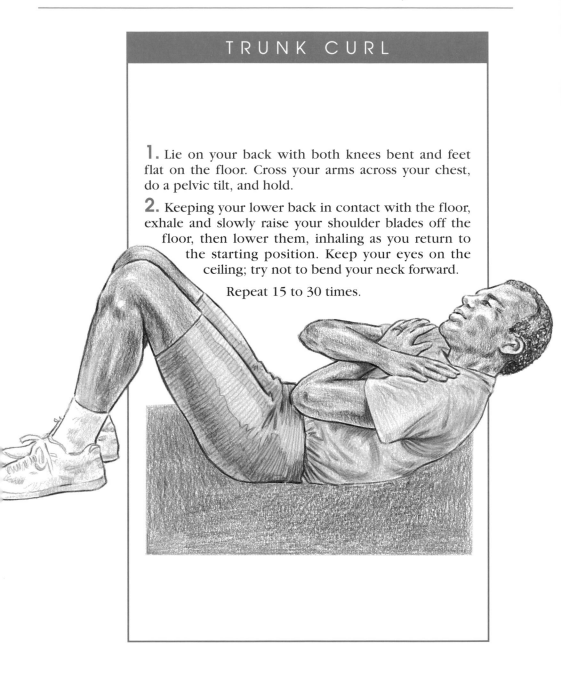

PRESS UP

1. Lie facedown on the floor with your hands by your shoulders.

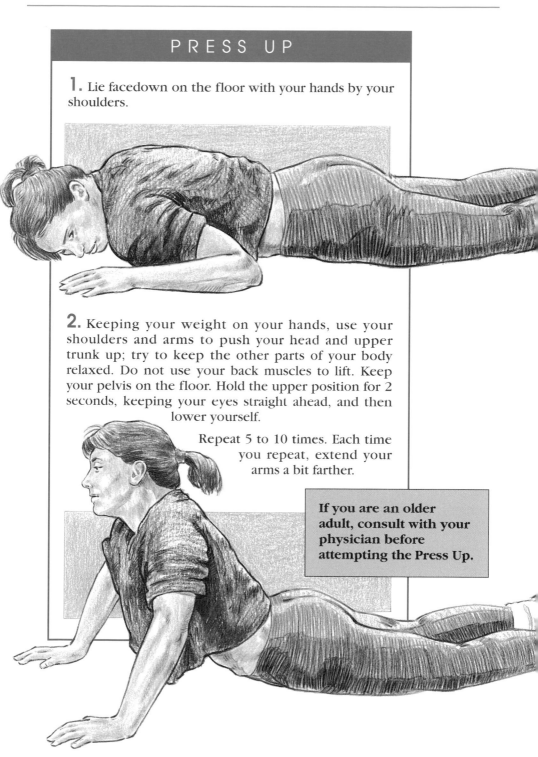

2. Keeping your weight on your hands, use your shoulders and arms to push your head and upper trunk up; try to keep the other parts of your body relaxed. Do not use your back muscles to lift. Keep your pelvis on the floor. Hold the upper position for 2 seconds, keeping your eyes straight ahead, and then lower yourself.

Repeat 5 to 10 times. Each time you repeat, extend your arms a bit farther.

If you are an older adult, consult with your physician before attempting the Press Up.

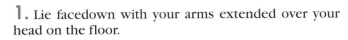

PRONE EXTENSION

1. Lie facedown with your arms extended over your head on the floor.

2. Exhale, slowly lift your left arm and right leg 6 to 12 inches (about 15 to 30 centimeters) off the floor, and hold for 3 to 5 seconds. Keep your eyes on the floor. Do not hold your breath. Lower your arm and leg, then do the same exercise using your right arm and left leg.

Repeat 10 to 15 times per pair.

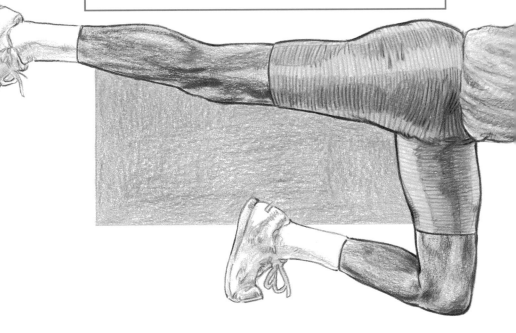

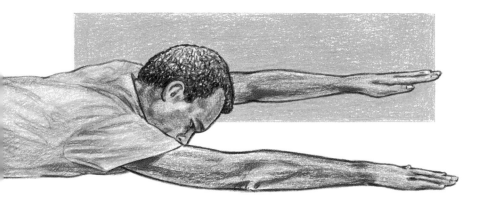

Level 3

Again, move to exercises in this level only after you arc able to do the maximum number of repetitions and hold for the maximum amount of time for most of the Level 2 exercises. You are continuing to condition the muscles that support your back.

QUADRUPED (ADVANCED)

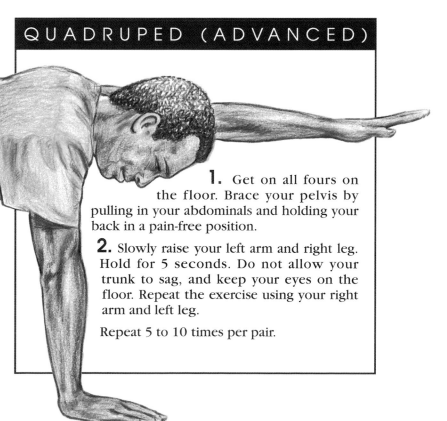

1. Get on all fours on the floor. Brace your pelvis by pulling in your abdominals and holding your back in a pain-free position.

2. Slowly raise your left arm and right leg. Hold for 5 seconds. Do not allow your trunk to sag, and keep your eyes on the floor. Repeat the exercise using your right arm and left leg.

Repeat 5 to 10 times per pair.

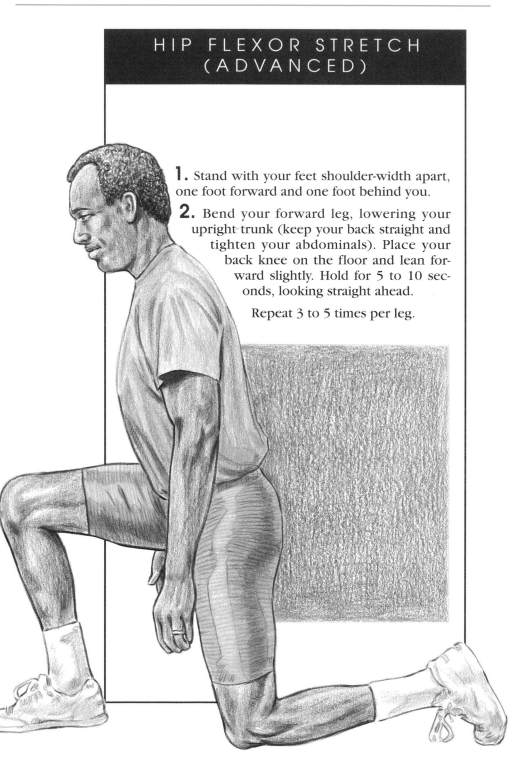

HIP FLEXOR STRETCH (ADVANCED)

1. Stand with your feet shoulder-width apart, one foot forward and one foot behind you.

2. Bend your forward leg, lowering your upright trunk (keep your back straight and tighten your abdominals). Place your back knee on the floor and lean forward slightly. Hold for 5 to 10 seconds, looking straight ahead.

Repeat 3 to 5 times per leg.

LOWER TRUNK ROTATION

1. Lie on your back with both knees bent and feet flat on the floor. Extend your arms out to your sides.

2. Slowly bring both knees toward your chest.

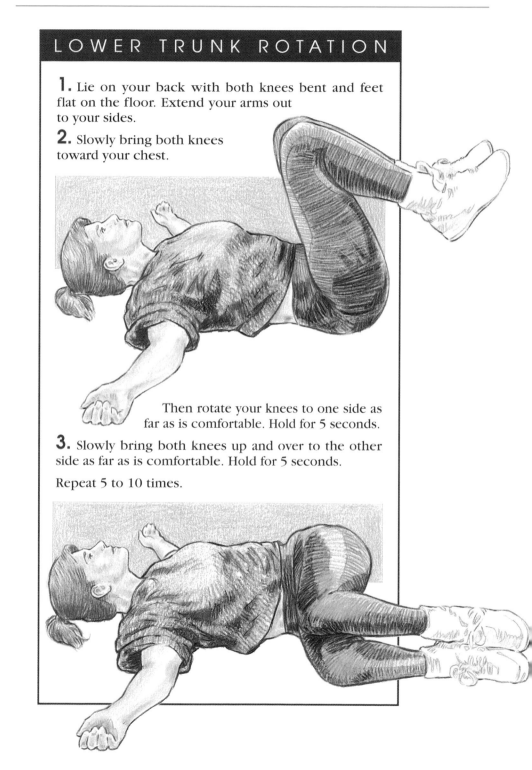

Then rotate your knees to one side as far as is comfortable. Hold for 5 seconds.

3. Slowly bring both knees up and over to the other side as far as is comfortable. Hold for 5 seconds.

Repeat 5 to 10 times.

SINGLE LEG RAISE (ADVANCED)

1. Lie on your back with both legs straight (or with both knees bent if you are uncomfortable when your legs are straight) and arms at your sides. (You may wish to place a small pillow under your head or neck.) Do a pelvic tilt and hold.

2. Keeping your lower back in contact with the floor, slowly raise one extended leg as high as possible without pain. (Do not point or flex your foot.) After you have raised your leg as far as you can, keeping your knee straight but not locked, gently pull your leg closer to you as you contract the front of your thigh. Hold for 10 seconds.

Repeat 5 to 10 times per leg. Your goal should be to raise each leg a minimum of 80 degrees off the floor; the position of your pelvis makes this more difficult than the earlier exercise *if* both legs are straight when you start raising one leg.

DIAGONAL CURL

1. Lie on your back with both knees bent, feet flat on the floor, and arms at your sides.

2. Exhale, and lift your trunk slightly. While lifting, rotate your trunk slightly by reaching both arms toward the right side of your right knee, lifting your left shoulder off the floor (your right shoulder may still be in contact with the floor). Look at your hands.

3. Inhale, and lower your shoulder and head to the floor, then do the same to the left side.

Repeat 10 to 15 times per side. For variation, reduce the number of repetitions but hold your right or left position by contracting your abdominals for 5 to 15 seconds.

Be sure to continue doing trunk curls from Level 2 frequently so you work all of your abdominal muscles.

SUPINE BRACING

1. Lie on your back with your legs straight. Place your hands on your lower abdominals and pull them in, then do a pelvic tilt and hold.

2. Keeping your lower back in contact with the floor, bring your right leg toward your chest while lifting your left leg off the floor. (Your left leg will be kept straight.) Then do the reverse, bringing your left leg toward your chest while straightening your right. Be sure you keep your abdominals tight and your lower back on the floor.

Repeat 10 to 20 times per leg.

If you must restrict your activity due to a cardiac condition, then do not perform Supine Bracing because this exercise requires strong isometric contraction (i.e., contraction against resistance) of your trunk muscles.

UPPER TRUNK RAISE

1. Lie facedown on the floor, arms at your sides.

2. Slowly elevate your head and shoulders from the floor. Raise them only to the point where you feel comfortable; don't force it. Look straight ahead. Hold for 5 to 10 seconds.

Repeat 5 to 10 times.

Don't exceed the normal standing curvature of your lower back.

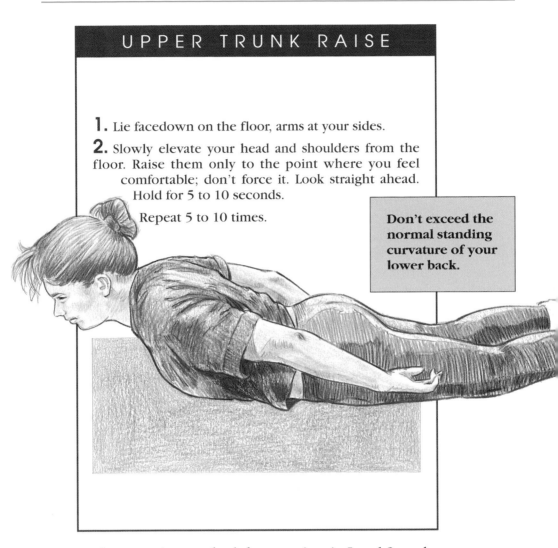

Once you've reached the exercises in Level 3, make them part of your regular exercise regimen at least three times a week. To preserve the gains you've made, you need to continue with these exercises from now on. You may want to go back to earlier exercises occasionally to check whether the muscles used in those movements are becoming weaker or stiffer and would benefit from your performing those exercises again.

Aerobic Exercise

If you do Level 3 exercises regularly, your back should feel better and you should be less likely to have a recurrence of back pain. But why stop there? You can do both your back and the rest of your body a favor by getting into a regular routine of aerobic exercise as well. *Aerobic exercise* is any rhythmic exercise that uses large muscle groups (such as the legs and arms), places demands on your heart and lungs, and can be performed at moderate intensity.

Keeping exercise at moderate intensity is important, because it's best to exercise continuously for at least 20 to 30 minutes if you want to condition your heart and lungs. But even shorter periods of exercise will have some effect, so, as far as your body is concerned, some exercise is better than none!

General fitness has been shown to correlate with less back pain, with the most fit people having the least trouble. Two possible reasons for this are

- it conditions you and your back-support muscles, and

- it keeps off extra pounds.

Aerobic exercise is one of the easiest ways to lose unwanted weight. It burns calories, and it also helps your body burn more fat and less lean tissue. We'll talk more about weight control in chapter 6.

If you don't already participate in an aerobic activity, check with your physician before you begin, then select one that appeals to you. If you're not sure about what you might like, try several—there are many to choose from. Some good beginning activities include

- walking,

- riding a bicycle (stationary or regular), and

- swimming.

These low-impact activities don't stress the spine much, and they allow you to start out gently. For sample starter programs and guidance on how to set up a complete fitness program, take a look at the *ACSM Fitness Book*. Written by the American College of Sports Medicine, it presents the basics of overall fitness and how to achieve it.

Check with your local YMCA or other fitness facility to see what aerobic activities they offer. Most have a variety of choices, from swimming classes to low-impact aerobics.

Strength Training

Strength training, if done carefully, can help condition your supporting back muscles and build bone strength. If you're interested in learning strength-training exercises, call your local fitness facility to see if they have a strength-training program. Let the local instructor know about your back problems so he or she can help you find the safest way to work out.

Another resource for strength training is *Weight Training: Steps to Success* by Thomas R. Baechle and Barney R. Groves and its partner video *Weight Training Video: Steps to Success*.

Aquatic Back Exercises

After trying out the previous back exercises, you may have found they were just what you needed. If you have other medical problems or conditions, though, such as arthritis or obesity, you might consider an alternative form of exercise—aquatic back exercise. You might want to try these just as a break from your regular land exercises, too, especially if swimming is already part of your schedule.

Exercising in the water has several advantages. The water's buoyancy lessens the stress on weight-bearing joints, making movement more comfortable. The water also provides mild resistance to all movements, gently working your muscles. And when the water is warm, it's easier to relax your muscles, which aids in stretching.

As with land exercises, don't continue doing an aquatic exercise if it is painful. Check with a medical professional to see if it's all right for you to perform the exercise before you try it again. All the precautions listed on pages 36–37 still apply here.

Here are a few aquatic back exercises to get you going:

WARM-UP

1. Walk in chest-deep water for 5 minutes. For variety, try walking in these and other ways: step high with good posture, holding your head high; walk forward, heel-toe, heel-toe; walk backward, toe-heel, toe-heel.

2. Squat down so your shoulders are underwater. In a circular motion, lift your shoulders up toward your ears, then move your shoulders forward and downward. Do 5 to 20 repetitions.

3. Reverse the shoulder-roll direction and do 5 to 20 repetitions.

Don't overdo the following exercises. Start with 5 repetitions and gradually work up to doing 20.

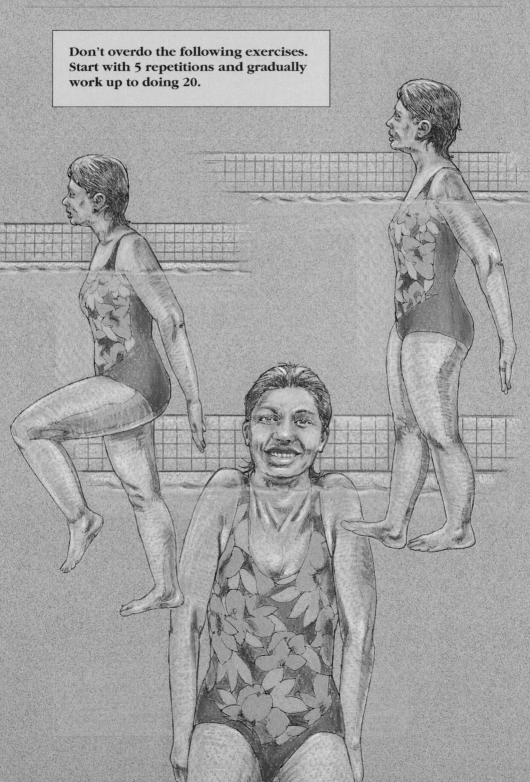

ARM RAISES

1. Stand with your back to the pool wall, feet 6 to 8 inches (about 15 to 20 centimeters) from the wall.

2. Keep your arms at your sides and submerge your shoulders. With your palms up, raise your arms in front of you to shoulder level. Then, with your palms down, lower your arms to your thighs.

Repeat 5 to 20 times.

ARM CROSSES

1. With your arms straight out in front at shoulder level, cross your arms in front of you.

2. Open them to the sides, and cross the opposite way. For more resistance, turn your palms toward each other for the inward movement and away from each other for the outward movement.

Repeat 5 to 20 times.

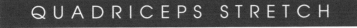

QUADRICEPS STRETCH

1. With your right side to the pool wall, start with your left knee lifted toward your chest. Hold on to the pool wall with your right hand for balance.

2. Hold your knee with your left hand, and while you slide your hand toward your ankle, slowly point your knee toward the pool floor until you feel a stretch in the front of your thigh. Do not arch your back. Hold the stretch for 5 to 10 seconds.

Repeat 5 to 20 times, then switch legs.

CALF STRETCH

1. Face the pool wall and hold on to it for balance. Put your right leg forward, knee bent, and your left leg backward, straight with your foot flat.

2. Keeping your back straight and buttocks tucked under, look toward the pool wall and lean toward it until you feel a stretch in your left calf. Hold for 5 to 10 seconds.

Repeat 5 to 20 times, then switch legs.

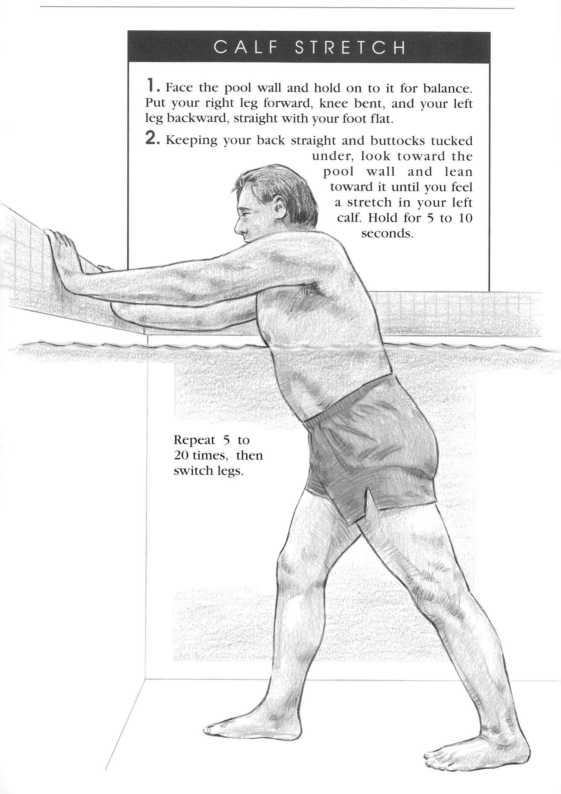

HAMSTRING STRETCH

1. Facing the pool wall, place your left toes on the wall at the junction of the pool wall and the floor, and stand with your right foot under the hips. Keep your back straight and hold on to the pool wall for balance.

2. Looking toward the pool wall, bend forward at your hip and bend your right knee until you feel a stretch at the back of your left thigh. Hold the stretch for 5 to 10 seconds.

Repeat 5 to 20 times, then switch legs.

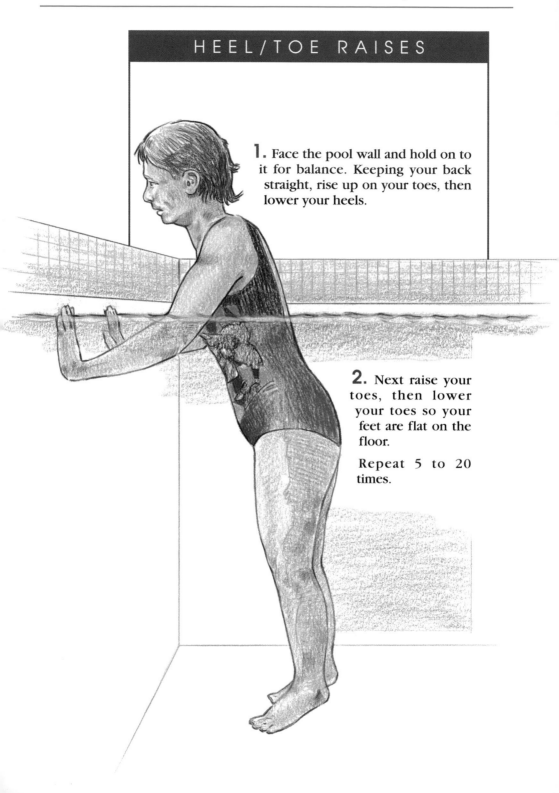

HEEL/TOE RAISES

1. Face the pool wall and hold on to it for balance. Keeping your back straight, rise up on your toes, then lower your heels.

2. Next raise your toes, then lower your toes so your feet are flat on the floor.

Repeat 5 to 20 times.

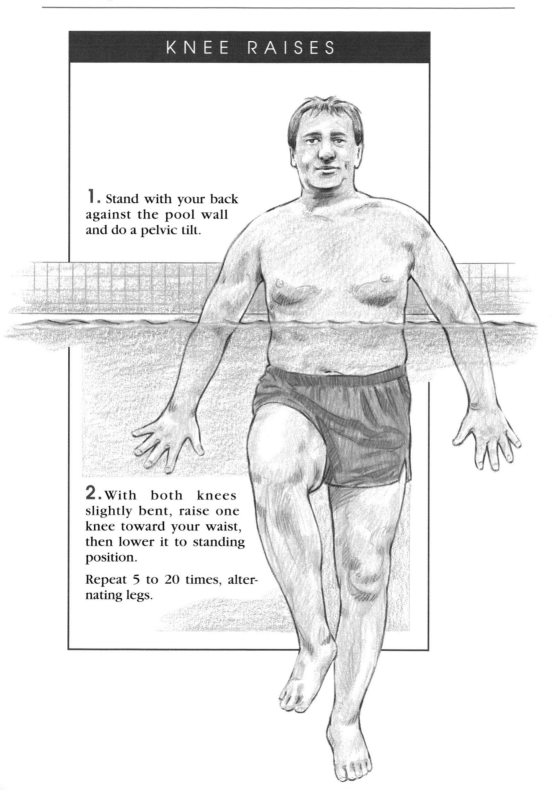

KNEE RAISES

1. Stand with your back against the pool wall and do a pelvic tilt.

2. With both knees slightly bent, raise one knee toward your waist, then lower it to standing position.

Repeat 5 to 20 times, alternating legs.

SLIDES

1. Stand with your back against the pool wall, feet shoulder-width apart, and heels 12 to 18 inches (about 30 to 46 centimeters) from the wall.

2. In pelvic tilt position (back flat, buttocks tucked under), bend your knees and slide down the wall slowly, hold for 3 seconds, then slide up. Don't bend your knees more than 90 degrees.

Repeat 5 to 20 times.

AEROBIC ACTIVITIES

After performing the back exercises, try some mild aerobic activity such as water walking or deep-water jogging.

Keep your back straight to avoid low back pain.

To water walk, simply walk through water at least 3-1/2 feet (about 1 meter) deep. The deeper the water, the more resistance you will encounter and the harder you will have to work. Deep-water jogging requires some type of flotation device to suspend you as you jog in place in water deep enough that your feet don't touch bottom. Ask an aquatics fitness instructor to recommend the best flotation device to use.

As you become more familiar with exercise in the water, you may want to pursue swimming. Work with an aquatics instructor to learn proper stroke techniques, and use only those strokes that don't hurt your back.

By exercising, whether on land or in the water, you will help prevent back pain and discomfort. But there are some additional steps you can take to protect your back. Being aware of a few key points about movement during daily tasks can help you perform those tasks with less stress on your back.

CHAPTER 5

Working With Your Back–Not Against It

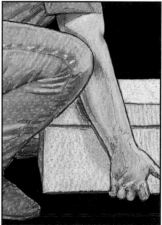

Our habits of movement—how we sit at our desks, how we lift the baby out of the playpen, how we sit when we drive, even how we sleep—affect our backs. Without realizing it, we can irritate or fatigue our back or neck muscles as we go about our tasks.

Relearning how to do the daily tasks of life isn't always easy, but it can pay off by reducing or avoiding back pain. Good posture is essential no matter what we do, and we can find ways to lessen the stresses in both sedentary and active work.

Good Posture

Hearing about good posture may take you back to the good old days when your mom told you to "Sit up straight." Or it may remind you of the military's command to "Stand at attention, chin in, chest out, stomach tight." Even though neither of these depicts good posture as either comfortable or pleasant, keeping your body correctly aligned can, in fact, lessen stress on your back and make you look more attractive in the process.

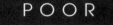

POOR

Your head is forward, your lower back is extended, and your stomach is out. Your shoulders and hips are uneven.

GOOD

Your shoulders are held so your arms fall naturally at your sides, your fingers along your pants seam. Your head is held erect, your chin is tucked in gently. Draw a line through your ear, center of torso, and leg. Your shoulders and hips are even.

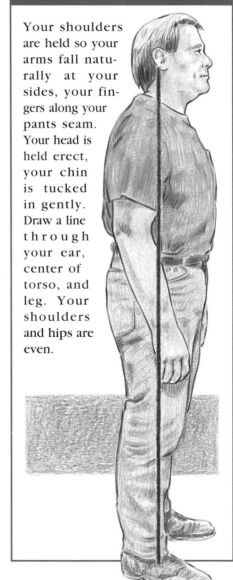

If you want to check your own posture, you'll need the following:

- A length of string or rope that will reach from ceiling to floor
- A tack or tape
- A camera and film (preferably Polaroid, so you get immediate feedback)
- Someone to take your picture

Hang the string or rope from the ceiling. Stand next to it sideways so the string or rope is next to your ear. Have your helper take your picture, then compare it with the preceding good and poor posture examples and note how they differ.

Now that you know how to stand with good posture, here are a few more tips on using correct posture during your daily activities.

While each activity requires a slightly different approach, these two rules apply across the board:

1. Try to maintain the normal curve of your lower back (whatever the normal curve is for you).

   - Tighten your abdominal muscles and don't slouch.

   - Keep your knees slightly higher than your hips when sitting; elevate one foot when standing.

   - Use a lower back support (a towel or small pillow) when sitting.

2. Don't stay in one position for a long time. Get up from whatever you're doing to move and stretch.

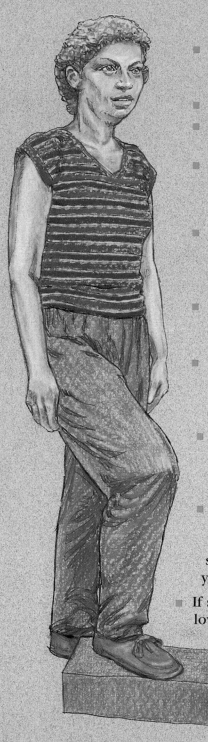

When you stand . . .

- If you can, elevate one foot slightly on a stool or box. Shift your feet from time to time.
- Shift your weight often.
- If you are carrying a bag, shift it from one shoulder to the other.
- If you wear high heels and have back trouble, try wearing lower heeled shoes.

When you sit . . .

- Sit slightly reclined, your knees higher than your hips, with your lower back supported. Your feet should be flat on the floor or on a footrest.
- To move closer to work on a desk or table, move your chair in. Don't move your head forward.
- Don't slump. If you are sitting in a soft chair or sofa and find it hard to keep from slumping, put a small pillow or towel behind your lower back.
- Get up and move around every 20 to 30 minutes.

When you sleep . . .

- Sleep either on your back, with your head low and a small pillow or rolled towel under your knees, or on your side, perhaps with a pillow between your knees.
- If sleeping on your stomach stresses your lower back, place a small pillow under your stomach to keep your lower back from sagging.
- Use a firm mattress, which will provide good support and make you change position more often as you sleep.

When you drive . . .

- Keep your back against the seat, using a lower back support if needed.
- Keep your body close to the steering wheel.
- Move the seat up so your feet are close enough to easily reach the pedals. Don't stretch your legs out.
- Stop frequently to get out and move around.
- Try not to jump into strenuous activity just after a long car trip. The vibrations from the car fatigue your back muscles.
- To get into the car, stand with your back to the car, placing one hand on the door and one on the seat back. Sit down gently. Bend your hips and knees to lift both feet onto the car's ledge. Use your hands to help turn your entire body forward in the seat.

Sitting Down on the Job

At first glance, sedentary work would appear to be easier for your back than manual labor. There's no heavy lifting, and you aren't twisting and turning much. But sitting much of the day takes its toll by weakening muscles, and when you already have trouble with your back, bad posture can aggravate it.

Be sure to take frequent stretch breaks from your work. Set your watch alarm as a reminder, or take stretch breaks at natural breaks in your work. In addition, follow these guidelines for working at your desk or computer:

When at your computer . . .

- Adjust the height of the chair or computer stand so the top of the computer screen is slightly below eye level.
- Position the computer directly in front of you (not to the side).
- Keep the front of the screen approximately one arm's distance away, and tilt it to avoid glare.
- Use an adjustable holder for any copy.
- Make sure you are getting both lumbar and forearm-wrist support.
- Use a footrest if it feels comfortable or if you need one.

When at your desk . . .

- Make sure your chair provides good lumbar support.
- Sit up straight.
- Keep your body close to the desk.
- Use a slantboard to hold any copy placed on the desk.
- Rest your forearms on the desk or on the arms of the chair.
- Use a footrest to raise your knees slightly above your hips.
- If curving forward feels good for your back, you can lean on the desk, using your arms to support your trunk (a tripod position of sorts).

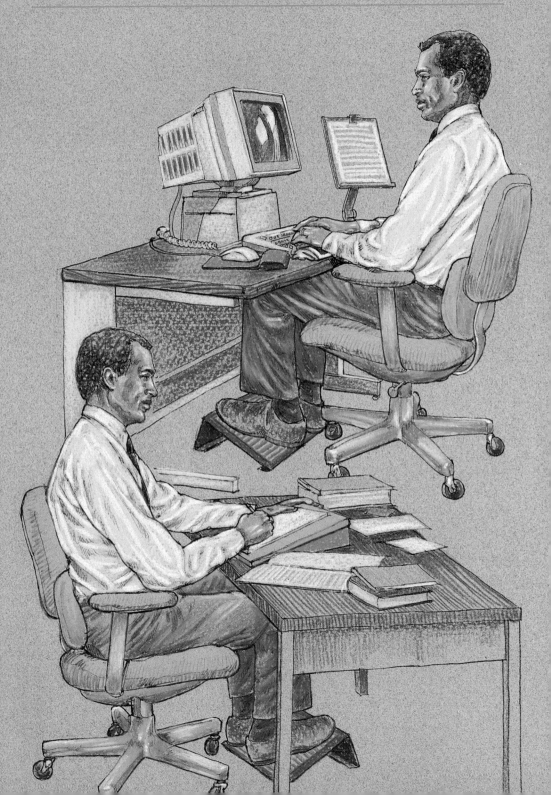

When in your ideal chair . . .

- Make sure the chair's seat pad offers good thigh support and adequate space on either side of your body so you can move around easily.

- Notice whether or not the armrests are adjustable and are close enough to not require leaning.

- Be able to tilt the chair's back slightly (at least 10 degrees), but not too far. Note if the chair's back is high enough and wide enough to support your back (it should be slightly wider than your torso and just below your shoulders), and if it provides adjustable lumbar support—ask your doctor to recommend the best one for you.

- Make sure the chair's frame turns easily and has casters.

Taking On Physical Tasks

One of the few things back pain researchers agree on is that lifting or moving objects adds stress to your back, particularly when combined with bending, twisting, reaching, moving suddenly, or when the objects are heavy. It pays to be cautious when performing these activities, even if they normally don't cause you pain.

You probably can protect your back in many daily situations by keeping these three principles in mind:

1. Whenever you need to reach down, bend your knees to keep from bending at your waist. This puts less stress on your back muscles and more on your stronger leg muscles.

   - If you have to bend at your waist, support yourself on surrounding structures with one or both arms.

   - Avoid bending at your waist by instead squatting or kneeling on one or both knees.

2. When lifting or moving objects, keep them as close to the middle of your body as possible. Think of your arms as a lever. The farther away from your body the object you're holding is, the more force it will put on your back.

   - Bend your knees to lower your body to the object (unless doing so prevents you from getting the object close to your body).

   - Stand on a stool to raise your body to the object.

   - Remove or go around obstacles between you and the object (for instance, the side of a pickup truck).

3. When standing to work, keep your hip flexed.

   - Put one foot up on a stool or box as you work, and switch feet often.

Follow the next few tips for performing specific daily chores and work activities to keep your back healthy and pain-free.

Lifting

Three common situations in which lifting occurs are lifting objects from the floor, from a shelf, and from inside a box, a car trunk, or other recessed area.

Avoid twisting or rotating as you lift and, whatever you do, try not to jerk the load you are lifting.

From a Shelf . . .

- Stand on a stool.
- Bend your knees.
- Don't reach way above your head and don't stand on your tiptoes.

From a Trunk . . .

- Put one knee on the bumper *or* extend one leg backward.
- Hold on to the side of the car with one hand.
- Get the object as close to your body as you can before lifting.

From a Crib . . .

- Place one leg on a footstool.
- Put the side of the crib down and lean your forearms on the edge.
- Get the child as close to your body as you can before lifting.

From the Floor . . .

- Evaluate the object and ask someone to help you if it looks heavy.
- Bend at your knees, not at your waist, and straddle the object to be lifted.
- Tuck your pelvis under and tighten your abdominal muscles.
- Keep the object you are lifting close to your body.
- Let your leg muscles do the work; feel them tighten as you lift.

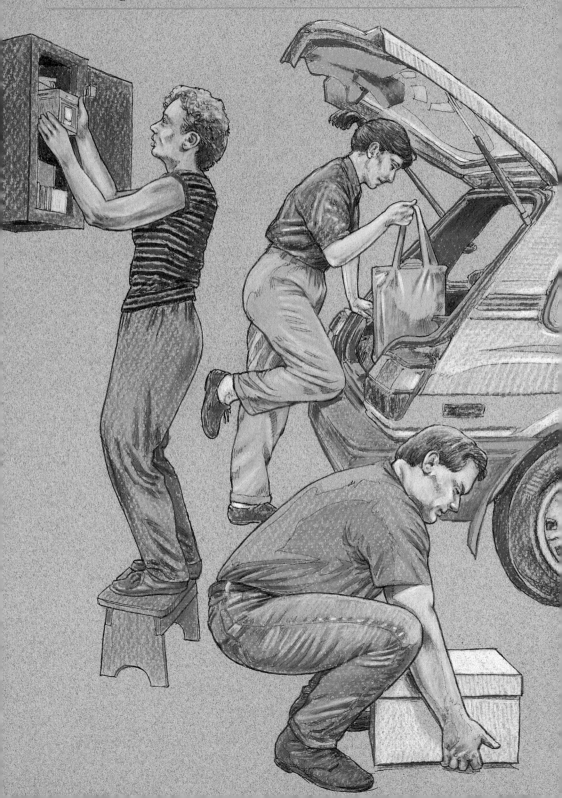

Pushing and Pulling

Always push, don't pull. Pushing, especially with your knees bent, uses your stomach and leg muscles more and your back muscles less. It also puts less pressure on your back.

Bending Over to Work

Whenever possible, avoid bending over to work; instead, kneel, either on one knee or both, or bend your knees and stoop.

Standing to Work

It's easy to fatigue your lower back when you stand for long periods of time to cook, iron, or do other tasks. Get a stool or box to put a foot up on, and switch feet from time to time.

Applying these movement techniques to your daily life can significantly reduce your chances of stressing or injuring your back. But there are other lifestyle issues you should also consider, ones that can lead to a healthier, less stressful way of life.

CHAPTER 6

A Healthy Lifestyle, A Healthy Back

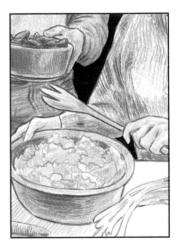

The final steps that you can take for your back are also steps that can improve your overall health. The first is to get or keep your weight under control; the second is to learn some form of relaxation you can use when tension worsens back pain.

Weight Control

If you are overweight, you probably aren't as fit as you should be. If some of your weight appears as an enlarged stomach, you may be putting additional stress on your back, especially since your stomach muscles are probably weak.

In addition, being obese—that is, having too much body fat—is not healthy. Heart disease and diabetes, as well as other diseases, are directly related to obesity.

83

It's also harder to exercise when you're carrying around more weight than you're comfortable with.

If you're ready to begin working on weight control, here are the basics of losing or maintaining weight.

Weight Loss

There is no magic way to lose weight. A calorie is a calorie is a calorie, no matter what kind of food it comes from. And you have to take in 3,500 calories a week less to lose 1 pound (0.45 kilogram) a week.

Don't be discouraged, though, because there are two ways to get rid of calories:

1. Eat fewer calories.

2. Exercise them away.

Depending on how much weight you need to lose, you can use just exercise or both exercise and changes in your diet to reach your goal. (It's not wise to just diet—more on that later.)

Weight loss should focus not necessarily on the number of pounds or kilograms but rather on the percentage of fat you have. Fat is the element that makes a difference in your health. Because muscle weighs more than fat, a muscular person may weigh more than normal according to height/weight charts, and yet be in good health.

Find Your Target Weight Range

Determining how much weight to lose is easy once you know your percentage of body fat. A professionally trained person can fairly accurately estimate your total body fat percentage by measuring the distance between skinfolds at set places on your body. The measurement is done with calipers and is not painful. With this measurement, the tester can help you determine your target weight range, the range of body weight that is appropriate for your good health.

If you don't have access to skinfold testing, you can use the following system from *Fitness Facts: The Healthy Living Handbook* by B. Don Franks and

Edward T. Howley to determine your target weight range. The only tools you'll need are a tape measure marked with inches and a bathroom scale that shows weight in pounds. (You may want to have a spouse or friend assist you in taking measurements.) The measurements you take will differ depending on whether you are a man or a woman.

Start by taking measurements and finding your percentage of body fat.

Find your percentage of body fat . . .

If you are a woman

- Measure your standing height (without shoes) in inches.

- Measure around your hips at the widest point in inches.

- Draw a straight line from your hip measurement on the left vertical line to your standing height on the right vertical line.

- Find the point on the middle vertical line where the line you drew crosses. That is your estimated percent body fat.

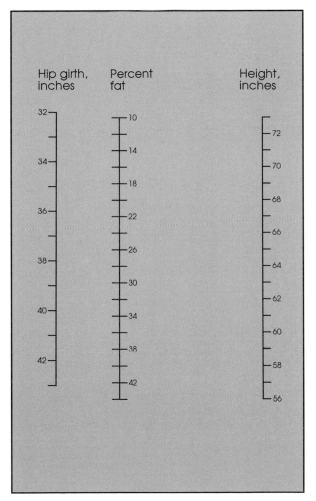

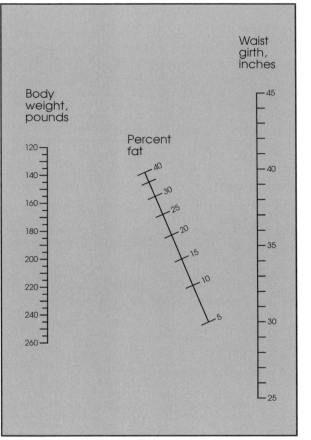

Complete the form on p. 87 to calculate your target weight range.

If you are a man

- Determine your weight in pounds.

- Measure your waist at the widest point in inches.

- Draw a straight line from your body weight on the left vertical line to your waist measurement on the right vertical line.

- Find the point on the middle diagonal line where the line you drew crosses. That is your estimated percent body fat.

Diet Sensibly

A reasonable rate of weight loss is 1/2 to 2 pounds (0.23 to 0.91 kilograms) a week. You may think that a starvation diet (900 calories or less daily) is a good idea because it works faster, but think again.

If you lose weight too fast, you lose muscle tissue as well as fat. Because muscle tissue burns more calories than fat, your efforts are counterproductive. And on

> Avoid starvation diets because a diet that is too low in calories causes your metabolism, the rate at which your body burns calories, to actually slow down. So you end up using fewer calories than you normally would. This effect even continues for some time *after* you diet.

Calculating Target Weight Range

1. Weigh yourself to get your current body weight: _____ pounds

2. Record your percent body fat: _____ %

3. Multiply your percent body fat, converted to a decimal value, by your body weight to yield fat weight:

   Body fat 0.____ x body weight _____ pounds = _____ pounds fat weight

4. Subtract this fat weight from your total body weight (Number 1) to yield lean weight:
   Body weight _____ pounds – fat weight _____ pounds = _____ pounds lean weight

5. If you are a woman, divide your lean weight by .81 to .77 (19% to 23% body fat). If you are a man, divide your lean weight by .84 to .80 (allowing for 16% to 20% ideal body fatness).(Remember that 84% lean weight corresponds to 16% fat weight; 80% lean weight, 20% fat weight; and so forth.)

Women

Lean weight _____ pounds ÷ .81 = _____ pounds

Lean weight _____ pounds ÷ .77 = _____ pounds

Target weight range is _____ pounds

Men

Lean weight _____ pounds ÷ .84 = _____ pounds

Lean weight _____ pounds ÷ .80 = _____ pounds

Target weight range is _____ pounds

For example:

- If a man is 24% fat and weighs 189 pounds, his fat weight is 45.4 pounds (.24 times 189 pounds = 45.4 pounds).
- Subtracting 45.4 pounds from 189 pounds leaves 143.6 pounds of lean weight.
- His ideal body fatness range is 16% to 20%, so divide 143.6 pounds by .84 and by .80 to yield 171 to 179.5 pounds as his target weight range.

top of that, when you start to eat normally again, your body will regain fat more easily than muscle. You may end up with more fat than you started with!

If you diet, then gain, over and over again, your metabolism slows even more, and weight loss becomes even harder. This "yo-yo" dieting can be worse than staying at your original weight. So what's the answer?—exercise, nutrition, and changing your eating behaviors.

Exercise

Research has shown that those who are most success-ful at taking weight off are those who exercise. Why?

1. Exercise burns additional calories.

2. Exercise builds muscles, which, even during rest, require more calories than fat.

3. Weight lost by dieting alone, without exercise, is 35% to 45% lean tissue, not fat.

4. Increased aerobic fitness makes muscles more able to burn fat.

We talked about exercise in chapter 4. Getting aerobic exercise at least three times a week is good for your health; if you want to lose weight more quickly, you can gradually work up to as many as six times a week.

Besides setting aside time for exercise, you can also change your daily routine to help burn more calories. Walk short distances rather than taking the car; go up the stairs rather than waiting for the elevator. Moving your body helps, whether it's labeled as exercise or not!

Nutrition

If the amount of weight you have to lose goes beyond what you can eliminate by exercise alone, or if you want to lose it a bit more quickly, then you need to watch your daily nutrition habits—not "diet."

For good health, you should eat a number of serv-ings from each food group daily.

Daily Nutrition

Food groups	What counts as a serving?	Number of servings per day
Bread, cereal, rice, and pasta	1 slice of bread; 1 ounce of ready-to-eat cereal; 1/2 cup of cooked cereal, rice, or pasta	6-11
Vegetable	1 cup of raw leafy vegetables; 1/2 cup of other vegetables, cooked or chopped raw; 3/4 cup of vegetable juice	3-5
Fruit	1 medium apple, banana, or orange; 1/2 cup of chopped, cooked, or canned fruit; 3/4 cup of fruit juice	2-4
Milk, yogurt, and cheese	1 cup of milk or yogurt; 1-1/2 ounces of natural cheese; 2 ounces of processed cheese	2-3
Meat, poultry, fish, dry beans, eggs, and nuts	2 to 3 ounces of cooked lean meat, poultry, or fish; 1/2 cup of cooked dry beans, 1 egg, or 2 tablespoons of peanut butter also count as 1 ounce of lean meat	2-3

One key to losing weight is to cut fat out of your diet as much as possible. Dietary fat is problematic in two ways:

1. It has 9 calories per gram, unlike carbohydrates and protein that have only 4 calories per gram.

2. The body expends less energy to convert fat calories into body fat than carbohydrate calories. Fat makes fat!

Many fats also raise blood cholesterol levels, which can cause heart disease.

> **Avoid saturated fats, found in meat, dairy products, eggs, and coconut and palm oils—they *raise* cholesterol.**
>
> **Use polyunsaturated fats, found in vegetable oils and some fish, and monounsaturated fats, as in olive, peanut, and canola oils—they *lower* cholesterol.**

Besides following these guidelines, you can lose weight and improve your health by eating less of these things:

- Sugar and alcohol—These have empty calories that have no nutritional value. Sugar also contributes to tooth decay.

- Salt—Too much salt has been linked to high blood pressure and heart disease for some people.

Eat more foods that contain these:

- Fiber—Foods with fiber usually reduce the amount of calories you eat, possibly by making your stomach feel full. Fiber also helps reduce cholesterol and may protect against some gastrointestinal diseases.

- Calcium—Sufficient calcium intake now helps prevent osteoporosis later. It is especially important for women to get enough calcium because they start out with less bone mass than men and lose bone rapidly after menopause. People 11 to 24 years old should take in 1,200 milligrams of calcium a day; after age 25 they only need 800 milligrams. Pregnant or lactating women should take in 1,200 milligrams daily.

Calcium-Rich Foods

Food groups	Excellent source (200–400 milligrams per serving)	Very good source (100–200 milligrams per serving)	Good source (50–100 milligrams per serving)
Dairy products	Low-fat yogurt, skim or low-fat milk, Swiss cheese, cheddar cheese, nonfat dry milk, tofu	Processed American cheese, cheese foods, cheese spread	Vanilla ice cream, cottage cheese
Seafood	Sardines (canned with bones)	Salmon (pink, canned with bones)	Clams (raw), oysters (raw), shrimp
Vegetables and fruit		Turnip greens, mustard greens, collard greens, dandelion greens, kale	Rhubarb, beet greens, spinach, okra, broccoli, almonds
Desserts		Custard (baked)	Pudding (made with low-fat milk)

Note. Most dairy products and foods made with dairy products (such as pizza and macaroni and cheese) have high calcium content. Though not actually dairy products, tofu and other soy products are often used as dairy substitutes.

Try these tips for cutting calories . . .

■ Choose lean meat, fish, poultry, dry beans, and peas as protein sources. Avoid fatty luncheon meats.

■ Trim excess fat off meats.

■ Broil, bake, or boil rather than fry.

■ Eat fewer creamed foods and rich desserts.

■ Limit your eating of highly processed foods, such as frozen foods or fast foods.

■ Drink skim or low-fat milk instead of whole milk.

- Use low-fat yogurt or cottage cheese in dips and dressings rather than sour cream, mayonnaise, or cream cheese.

- Choose cheeses made with skim or low-fat milk (mozzarella, Jarlsberg) rather than regular whole-milk cheeses (cheddar, Swiss).

- Instead of sweet snacks, try fruit or popcorn.

- Eat fruit instead of drinking fruit juice.

- Stay away from foods with labels that show sugar as the first or second ingredient.

- Cut back on the amount of sugar you use in recipes.

Behavioral Changes

Another way to help yourself control your weight is to become aware of your eating habits and find ways to change and control them. Then you'll want to reward yourself for it, too! Also enlist the help of your family and friends. Here are some suggestions to help make the changes easier.

Self-Monitoring

For at least a few weeks, keep an accurate record of everything you eat—snacks as well as regular meals. Be honest with yourself! Then look it over to see

- how much you actually eat,

- what situations trigger overeating, and

- what food substitutions you might try.

Make adjustments accordingly. You may also find that just the act of recording what you eat makes you change what or when you eat.

Strategies for Controlling Eating

Things in our environment may cue us to eat, even when we aren't necessarily hungry. The time of day (noon), the place (the kitchen), even the activity (watching TV) can get us started. To change these connections we've made, we need to try to delay, substitute, or avoid.

Delay

- Slow down the pace of eating.
- Do a relaxation exercise (see the next section of this chapter).
- Take the roundabout route to the kitchen.
- Preplan the purchase of tempting foods. Buy them in a form that needs a lot of preparation (like cake mix instead of a ready-made cake).
- Purchase snacks in individual packages so you have to open a new one each time you are considering a snack.
- Store tempting foods so they are difficult to get at.
- Put off unplanned eating as long as possible.

Substitute

Instead of eating, try one of these:
- Do a pleasant activity—walk, work in the garden, read, sleep.
- Do a necessary activity—run an errand, clean, make phone calls.

Avoid

- Minimize your contact with food. Try not to go near the kitchen at home or the eating area at work.
- Don't bring tempting foods into the house.
- If you can't stick to your diet when you eat with a particular person, try to avoid eating with him or her. Plan nonfood activities together.
- Spend your free time or coffee breaks away from food.
- Make food available only for meals and planned snacks.
- Make eating a single activity. Avoid eating as you do other things like reading the paper, watching TV, or driving.

- If you don't have to be in the kitchen when food is being prepared, get out.

- Ask other family members to prepare their own snacks and lunches.

- Store food in storage locations only, not in desk drawers, glove compartments, or nightstands.

- Serve meals from the kitchen or buffet. Avoid putting serving bowls on the table if possible. If foods are placed on the table during meals, set them out of your reach.

- Remove dishes as soon as possible after eating.

- Scrape food directly into the garbage or disposal after clearing.

- Wrap leftovers immediately after a meal and store them in the refrigerator or freezer.

- Incorporate leftovers into planned snacks or meals.

Self-Reward

Be sure to pat yourself on the back when you alter your eating behaviors. Any nonfood reward you promise yourself can help you stay on track. We'll give you some ideas here, but you might think of other rewards that would serve the same purpose.

Spend a little on yourself . . .

- Set aside a lump sum for when you reach a goal.

- Accumulate a bit each time you succeed, saving for a special purchase.

Break from your routine . . .

- Take a half day or full day to go shopping (not grocery shopping) for yourself.

- Go to a good movie or visit friends.

- Spend time on a favorite hobby.

- Read a book you've been wanting to read.

- Call a special friend who lives far away.

- Subscribe to a new magazine.

   Think positively . . .

- Congratulate yourself each time you succeed.

- Be proud of the progress you've made.

Social Support

Try to enlist the help of family and friends as you make changes in your eating habits. Ask them to encourage you (*not* nag) and to not offer you fattening foods or push you to eat. If they are willing, they might even reward you for your efforts, maybe giving you a back rub or doing the laundry.

Some people may become upset if you begin to take charge of your eating and lose weight. If they have wanted to lose weight themselves or they think you may become more attractive to others because you are thinner, it may threaten them. They may even try to sabotage your efforts by putting rich foods in your way and encouraging you to eat.

To help yourself and those around you, follow these tips:

■ *Be assertive*. State what you want and say no when you have to.

■ *Be open*. If you feel that someone is hurting your efforts, intentionally or otherwise, let him or her know—tactfully.

■ *Be specific*. Make it clear to others what you would like them to do to help you.

■ *Be consistent*. Don't give a mixed message by turning down something to eat one day and accepting it the next.

■ *Be positive*. Stay as enthusiastic as you can.

■ *Be thankful*. Tell those who help you how much you appreciate it.

Another form of social support might be taking a weight management class. Check with your local YMCA to see if it offers *Y's Way to Weight Management* classes or pick up Sandra K. Cotterman's book by the same name from which many of these suggestions were taken. Other fitness facilities may offer weight management classes as well.

Relaxation

Let's face it: We don't hurt as much when we're having a "good" day as we do on a "bad" one. Feeling stressed or upset can make pain feel worse. But we can learn to control stress by developing the skill of relaxation.

You may think you already know how to relax, that it's a natural state that's easy to achieve—but is that true? Take a moment right now and tighten the muscles in one arm briefly, then let them go. Compare how that arm feels with the opposite one. Does one feel more tense than the other? Does one feel warmer than the other? It's hard for us to be aware of where tension is unless we've trained ourselves to notice the differences between tension and relaxation. It's also hard, when we're already tense, to get a handle on how to let go. Practice helps us do it.

Many techniques for relaxation are possible. We'll offer a few here, and you can try each to see which works for you. Even if one doesn't work as well as you'd like, you still can find out more about how you experience relaxation and what triggers it for you.

Training Exercise

A good technique to begin with is this relaxation training exercise taken from Elizabeth Kirkaldy-Willis's chapter "The Back School" in *Managing Low Back Pain*. It helps you become aware of the differences between tension and relaxation and the places in your body that tend to become tense. When you tense parts of your body during the exercise, don't squeeze too hard, especially near any part of your body that is already painful. Tighten the muscles enough to feel them, but not enough to hurt.

1. Set aside 15 to 20 minutes of uninterrupted time. Use a quiet room away from a telephone, television, or other distractions. Loosen your clothing. Lie down with your hips and knees bent or sit with your knees higher than your hips.

2. Close your eyes or focus on a spot on the ceiling or wall. Concentrate and put all other things out of your mind.

3. Listen to your breathing. Concentrate on how smooth and regular it is. Place one hand just below your ribs. Your stomach should be rising and falling with your breathing. Continue to concentrate on your breathing. Take a slow, deep breath. As you breathe out, feel the tension going out of your body and feel yourself relax. Think of letting yourself become heavy and relaxed. Feel your stomach area slowly rise and fill like a balloon. Feel the air enter your nose and lungs. Let the air out slowly. Feel your stomach area gently fall. Feel yourself relaxing as you breathe out.

4. As you continue deep relaxed breathing you may start to feel pleasantly warm, and this is good. Improved blood circulation may raise your body temperature. Your legs and arms may feel heavy and relaxed. Try to remember this feeling. Teach your body to relax like this frequently during the day.

5. As you breathe in, tighten your right hand into a fist. Hold for 5 seconds, thinking, "My hand is tense." Then let your hand go limp for three to four breaths. Do this three times and then repeat with your left hand.

6. Tighten your right hand into a fist, bend your right elbow, and move your fist to your shoulder. At the same time, tighten your shoulder and neck muscles. Hold for 5 seconds, then relax for three to four breaths. Do this three times, and repeat with the left side.

7. Tighten and relax the muscles in your legs, back, and head one by one in the same way as just described.

8. Finish your relaxation session when you feel ready, but try to maintain some of that relaxed state as you open your eyes and get up.

This type of relaxation should be done often, daily if possible. Relaxing thoroughly is a skill, and it takes practice before you can do it well. You'll be amazed at how relaxed you can get after practicing it for 2 or 3 weeks.

If you have a chronic medical condition, especially one for which you take drugs, be sure to talk to your physician before doing regular relaxation exercises. Regular relaxation may cause healthy changes in your body that affect your treatment. If you take medicine for your condition, you may require an adjustment in the dosage.

It's also possible that you may experience some unusual emotional reactions as you become more relaxed. If they bother you, or if they continue for a long time, you may want to discontinue your relaxation practice or consider talking about your experiences with a trained counselor.

Once you've mastered the training exercise, you might want to develop some shorter ways to relax, ones that you can use at any time during the day when you need to cope with stress or pain.

Breathing

The breathing portion of the training exercise (Step 3) can be used by itself to help you calm yourself when things get stressful. When we're tense or excited, we tend to breathe quickly and shallowly, breathing primarily from the top part of the lungs. By consciously controlling breathing so it is slow, from deep within the lungs, and rhythmic, we can help reduce tension.

It may be more difficult for you to breathe this way if you smoke, have a tendency to hyperventilate (breathe too rapidly and shallowly), or usually have stomach or chest tension. With practice, though, most people can do it. If you have trouble, try using shorter breathing cycles and gradually lengthen them.

When you first try deep breathing, you may feel a bit light-headed. You may also find that when you breathe this way there is a longer than usual pause between breaths. These are signs that you are breathing more efficiently. A deep breath gets oxygen to your body much more effectively than a shallow one.

Visualization

Another quick method of inducing relaxation is visualizing a relaxing situation or location. When we imagine being in a pleasant place, our bodies will tend to react somewhat as if they were actually there. Thinking about lying on a beach under the hot sun usually makes our muscles release a bit, just as if we were being warmed by the sun. Visualization also temporarily takes us away from whatever problems we face, giving us a chance to calm down and enabling us to return to our work with a more balanced perspective.

If you want to try this, search your thoughts for several images that appeal to you. It could be a balmy beach in Hawaii, a cozy mountain cabin in the snow, or a favorite picnic spot. It could be floating in water or in the clouds or lying in a hammock. The image doesn't matter as long as there's nothing disturbing for you in it.

At the end of your training exercise, think about one of the images that you have chosen. Give it life by adding touches that appeal to your senses. For instance, if you imagine being on the beach by the ocean, can you hear the waves breaking on the shore? Can you feel the warm sun on your skin and the fine sand beneath you? Do seagulls soar across the sky?

You can then try thinking about that image during the day when you need a quick break. That mental vacation can be just what you need to stop the buildup of tension.

Develop more than one image so you can switch among them, depending on your mood. Using the same image over and over again can make it less powerful as time passes.

Cuing

Once you know how to relax, you can develop the ability to trigger relaxation quickly by using cuing. Cuing is simply choosing a word or phrase to link to your state of relaxation. A word often used is *relax*, but anything that makes sense to you will work.

What you need to do is pair the word or phrase with your state of relaxation. Whenever you relax, say the key word or phrase to yourself repeatedly. You may even find that a word doesn't work as well as a brief image or the act of beginning to breathe deeply. That's fine too.

Other Techniques

The techniques just discussed work well for most people, but if you feel they aren't what you need, or if you want to explore further, there are other possibilities. More active forms of relaxation, such as yoga, exercise, or T'ai Chi, may appeal to you. Self-hypnosis and autogenic training are other methods you might try.

This brings you to the end of the book, but to the beginning of a healthier lifestyle for you and your back. We've given you a lot of suggestions for protecting and conditioning your back daily. Try them a few at a time, choosing those you think would be most helpful first, and gradually make the changes that will reduce your chances of experiencing back pain. Start slowly with exercise, but make a commitment to do it. Seek support from family and friends—even have them read this book. After all, back pain will happen to most of us, sooner or later. You are not alone!

LUISA'S BACK STILL CAUSED HER PROBLEMS, but the pain was finally subsiding. She knew osteoporosis was serious, but instead of worrying, she focused on taking care of herself. She took her calcium and hormones daily, and three times a week she and Connie walked down to the Y together and went swimming. Actually, Luisa did her exercises and a little water walking, while Connie did all the swimming—she was becoming quite the little tadpole.

MIKE DIDN'T KNOW WHICH WAS WORSE, trying to stop smoking or trying to lose weight. Both seemed impossible at times, but with help from his wife he was beginning to make progress. He took out a stick of gum, opened his clipboard, and checked off each item as it was loaded by the guy with the forklift.

TRACY WASN'T ABOUT TO GIVE UP eating chocolate cake or watching great old movies, so, instead, she joined the Fit to Serve officer fitness program at work. She started out with a couple of light workouts a week, met a few people, and found a workout partner. Soon she was at the gym several times a week. She was in good shape and she felt great. She didn't even notice that her back pain was gone.

JAY'S JOB WAS GOING WELL—he'd landed three new accounts and the pressure from his boss was letting up. He was actually dealing with his stress. He put in fewer late nights at the office and spent more time with his family. At first he hated giving up his weekly games with the guys, but they could get rough, and, at 45, playing basketball with his kids was less painful and a lot more fun.

ACKNOWLEDGMENTS

Thanks go to the following people who served on the panel of experts who provided guidance and input for this book:

Dr. Wendell Liemohn
Professor
Department of Human Performance and Sport Studies
College of Education
The University of Tennessee, Knoxville, TN

Jeffrey A. Saal, MD
Sports, Orthopedic and Rehabilitation Medicine
    Associates
Menlo Park, CA

Lynne Vaughan
Associate Director for Health and Fitness
YMCA of the USA
Chicago, IL

Michael J. Spezzano
Corporate Program Director
YMCA of Greater New York
New York, NY

The exercises in chapter 4 were contributed by Dr. Liemohn, and we thank Sue Peterson for reviewing the section on office ergonomics.